# What about Becoming

# *A Caregiver*

# *in Radiology ?*

*MARTIN STERLING*

# Table of contents

« *Radiology is not just the art of seeing through, but the magic of deciphering the silent language of the body to guide the path to healing.* »

# INTRODUCTION

## The essential role of the nursing auxiliary in medical imaging

Medical imaging is a fascinating field that merges advanced technology with direct patient care. This combination requires a skilled medical team, in which the nursing auxiliary plays a crucial role. Their responsibilities, although often unknown to the general public, are fundamental to the smooth running of the radiology department and the well-being of the patient.

- First point of contact
    - Often, the healthcare assistant is the patient's first contact with the imaging department. This initial contact is crucial in establishing an atmosphere of trust. An empathetic and reassuring approach helps the patient to relax, which is essential for obtaining clear images and ensuring the patient's comfort.
    -
- Preparing the Patient
    - Before any imaging procedure, the patient often needs to be prepared. This may include explaining the process, changing into hospital clothes, checking medical history to ensure there are no contraindications to the examination (such as an allergy to the contrast medium), or even inserting a venous line. The nursing auxiliary is often in the front line for these tasks.

- Technical Assistance
  - Although the nursing auxiliary does not carry out the images themselves, they often assist the radiology technician or radiologist in various aspects of the procedure. This may include positioning the patient correctly, preparing equipment or administering contrast products under supervision.

- Safety and Radiation Protection
  - Safety is paramount in radiology. The care assistant must ensure that all safety protocols are followed, particularly with regard to radiation protection. This includes ensuring that the patient and staff are properly protected from unnecessary exposure to radiation.

- Post-examination care
  - After the examination, the role of the care assistant does not stop. They must ensure that the patient is well, provide post-examination care if necessary (such as monitoring a reaction to the contrast medium) and often provide instructions for follow-up.

- Liaison between the Patient and the Medical Team
  - The care assistant often acts as a bridge between the patient and the rest of the medical team, passing on crucial information that can influence patient care or the interpretation of images.

- Work Environment Maintenance
  - To ensure the safety and efficiency of the department, the care assistant is often involved in the general upkeep of the department, making sure that everything is clean, organised and functional.

The medical imaging assistant is an essential cog in the complex radiology machine. Without their dedication, skill and care, the imaging process would be far less fluid, efficient and humane.

# The fusion of skincare and technology: a unique combination

The world of medical imaging is a remarkable juxtaposition between human, patient-centred care and the use of cutting-edge technologies. This unique convergence makes it possible to obtain accurate diagnoses and targeted treatments, but it also requires a medical team that knows how to handle both sides of the coin.

- Technology: An Eye on the Invisible
  - **Diagnostic accuracy**: Technological advances in imaging allow doctors to see what was previously invisible. Whether it's a growing tumour, a vascular anomaly or a bone lesion, technology is giving us an unprecedented glimpse inside the human body.
  - **Minimising invasive procedures**: Thanks to medical imaging, many diagnoses and even some treatments can be carried out without the need for invasive surgical procedures. This reduces the risks to patients while speeding up their recovery.
  - **Constant evolution**: Imaging technology is evolving at a phenomenal rate. New imaging modalities and better resolutions mean that what we can see and how we see it is constantly improving.

- Care: The Human Behind the Machine
  - **Empathy and comfort**: Despite our dependence on technology, patient comfort and well-being remain paramount. An anxious or uncomfortable patient can affect the quality of the images. The empathetic approach of the care assistant and the medical team is therefore essential.
  - **Communication**: Explaining a procedure, reassuring a worried patient, or understanding an individual's specific needs are skills just as crucial as technical mastery of the equipment.
  - **Safety**: Although equipment can do a great deal, it is human vigilance and care that guarantee patient safety, whether in terms of protection against radiation or reactions to contrast agents.

- The Interdependence of Technology and Care
  - **Efficiency and Accuracy**: Without the human skill to position a patient correctly or to interpret the signals from a piece of equipment, the technology would lose its effectiveness.
  - **Personalised Care**: Despite the wonders of technology, every patient is unique. Adapting procedures, choosing the imaging modality, and making adjustments based on individual needs is a human decision.

- Continuing Education and Training
  - **Technological evolution**: As technology advances, the need for the medical team to stay informed and trained is paramount.
  - **Interpersonal skills**: Training in communication, stress management and patient interaction techniques is equally crucial

to ensuring that technology is used to best effect.

Although medical imaging relies heavily on technology, it is the fusion of this technology with attentive, patient-centred care that truly defines the field. It's a delicate dance, where machine and human complement each other to offer the best of both worlds in the service of the patient's well-being and health.

# Chapter 1:
# UNDERSTANDING RADIOLOGY

## History and development of radiology

Radiology, as a medical discipline, has come a long way since its accidental discovery at the end of the 19th century. Radiology's journey has been one of scientific curiosity, technological innovation and a growing understanding of its implications for health. Let's take a look at this fascinating story.

- The beginnings: Discovery of X-rays
  - **Wilhelm Conrad Röntgen (1895)**: This German physicist is credited with discovering X-rays while experimenting with cathode ray tubes. The image of the hand of his wife, Anna Bertha, is the first known X-ray.
  - **Initial reactions**: The discovery was greeted with wonder and scepticism. X-rays were used at fairs and exhibitions before finding a medical application.

- Early Development and Medical Use
  - **Early medical      uses**: Surgeons were quick to recognise the potential of X-rays for locating bullets and fractures. This was particularly useful during the wars to treat wounded soldiers.
  - **Realising the dangers**: Unfortunately, initial ignorance of the risks associated with radiation has led to a number of cases of over-exposure, some resulting in illness or even death.

- The Era of Modernisation and Specialisation
  - **Development of the Fluoroscope (1920s)**: This innovation enabled real-time visualisation, albeit still rudimentary.
  - **Tomography (1930s)**: Technique used to visualise specific sections of the body, improving the clarity and precision of images.
  - **Recognition as a Speciality**: Progress has solidified radiology as a distinct medical speciality requiring specialist training.

- Major Technological Innovations
  - **Computed tomography (CT) (1970s)**: A major advance, CT uses computers to create detailed cross-sectional images of the body.
  - **Magnetic Resonance Imaging (MRI) (1980s)**: Using magnetism and radio waves, MRI provides even more detailed images, particularly of soft tissue.
  - **Ultrasound**: Using sound waves to produce images, it is particularly useful for obstetrical and cardiac imaging.

- Interventional Radiology
  - This sub-field of radiology enables doctors to use imaging to guide minimally invasive procedures, whether for biopsies, vascular treatments or other interventions.

- Contemporary challenges and the future
  - **Radiation protection**: With a growing understanding of the risks, research continues into minimising radiation doses without compromising image quality.
  - **Artificial Intelligence and Radiology**: AI promises to increase diagnostic accuracy,

improve disease detection and personalise patient care.
- **Radiation-guided therapies**: Going beyond simple detection, radiology is playing a growing role in image-guided therapies to treat diseases directly.

Radiology is a field that illustrates the constant evolution of medicine. It began as a chance discovery and has evolved into a complex speciality that combines medical expertise and technological innovation for the benefit of patients around the world.

# The different medical imaging techniques

## • Standard radiography

Standard radiography, often referred to simply as "radiography", is the oldest and most commonly used form of medical imaging. It uses X-rays to obtain two-dimensional images of the inside of the body, enabling bones and certain organs to be visualised. Let's take a closer look at what standard radiography is, how it works, its applications, and its advantages and disadvantages.

- Fundamental principle
    - **Production of X-rays**: X-rays are produced when an electric current passes through an X-ray bulb, causing high-energy photons to be emitted.
    - **Differential Absorption**: X-rays pass through the body and are absorbed in different quantities depending on the density of the tissue. Bone, being denser, absorbs more X-rays and appears white on the X-ray. Less

dense tissues, such as muscles and organs, appear darker.

- Common Applications
  - **Bone examination**: to detect fractures, infections, tumours or congenital anomalies.
  - **Thoracic examination**: Assess the lungs, heart and other thoracic structures for infections, tumours or heart disease.
  - **Abdominal examination**: To visualise certain organs such as the stomach, intestines, liver or bladder.
  - **Dental check-up**: Assessment of the health of teeth and gums.

- Procedure
  - **Positioning**: The patient is positioned to obtain the optimum angle for the examination. This may require several shots from different angles.
  - **Radiation Protection**: Lead aprons can be used to protect certain parts of the body from unnecessary exposure to X-rays.

- Benefits
  - **Speed and accessibility**: X-rays are generally fast, which makes them particularly useful in emergencies.
  - **Cost**: Compared with other imaging modalities, radiography is relatively inexpensive.
  - **Ease of use**: Can be used in a wide range of environments, including hospitals, clinics and dental practices.

- Disadvantages and concerns
  - **Radiation exposure**: Although low, there is exposure to radiation. Clinicians always strive

to follow the ALARA (As Low As Reasonably Achievable) principle to minimise this exposure.
- **Image Limitation**: Radiography offers 2D images, which may limit the visualisation of certain anomalies or pathologies.

- Associated Technologies
  - **Digital radiography**: Instead of traditional film, images are captured electronically, offering improved viewing and handling.
  - **Fluoroscopy: A** form of real-time radiography, often used to guide medical procedures.

Standard radiography remains a cornerstone of diagnostic medicine. Although old in terms of medical technology, it continues to evolve and to play an essential role in patient care throughout the world.


## • Computed tomography (CT or scanner)

Computed tomography, also known as CT or CAT scan, is a medical imaging technique that uses X-rays to obtain detailed cross-sectional images of the body. Compared with standard X-rays, it offers much better resolution of detail, allowing doctors to see inside the body with unprecedented clarity. Let's delve into the fascinating world of CT.

- Fundamental principle
  - **Image acquisition**: CT uses a rotating X-ray beam to obtain images from different angles. The machine then combines these images to create detailed cross-sections of the body.

- **3D images**: By stacking transverse images, it is possible to reconstruct a three-dimensional image of the area of interest.

- The CT scanner
  - **X-ray Tube and Detectors**: These rotate around the patient to capture images from different angles.
  - **The Examination Table**: The patient lies on this table, which moves slowly through the scanner ring.
  - **The Control Console**: Used by technologists to control the scanner and view images.

- Common Applications
  - **Cerebral assessment**: Locating tumours, haemorrhages or vascular anomalies.
  - **Thoracic examination**: Detection of tumours, infections or lung diseases.
  - **Abdominal and Pelvic Study**: Assessment of organs such as the liver, kidneys, bladder and intestines.
  - **Angio-Scanner**: Visualisation of blood vessels and detection of abnormalities.
  - **Trauma assessment**: Precise location of injuries after an accident.

- Procedure
  - **Patient preparation**: Depending on the examination, a contrast agent may be administered to improve visualisation.
  - **Positioning**: The patient must remain still during the scan to obtain clear images.
  - **Duration**: Most CT scans are fast, often being completed in a few minutes.

- Benefits
  - **Anatomical details**: CT scans offer much higher resolution than standard X-rays.
  - **Flexibility**: It can be used to examine a wide variety of body structures.
  - **Guided procedures**: Scans can be used to guide biopsies or other procedures.

- Disadvantages and concerns
  - **Radiation exposure**: The radiation dose from a CT scan is generally higher than that from a standard X-ray, which is why clinical justification is so important.
  - **Allergic reactions**: Rarely, patients may react to the contrast material used during the scan.

- Technological developments
  - **Cone-beam CT**: Used mainly in dental imaging to obtain 3D images.
  - **Multi-slice scanners**: for faster image acquisition and higher resolution.
  - **AI applications**: Artificial intelligence is increasingly being integrated to improve disease detection and image accuracy.

Computed tomography is a powerful tool that has revolutionised diagnostic medicine. It is now essential in many fields, from neurology to trauma surgery, and continues to evolve thanks to technological advances.

## • Magnetic Resonance Imaging (MRI)

Magnetic Resonance Imaging, commonly known as MRI, is a medical imaging technique that uses powerful magnetic fields and radio waves to produce detailed images of the body's internal structures. It is distinguished by its absence of X-rays and its ability to finely differentiate soft tissue, making it indispensable in many medical fields.

- Fundamental principle
    - **Magnetic Resonance Phenomenon**: MRI exploits the fact that hydrogen nuclei in the human body (mainly in water) react when placed in a magnetic field. When stimulated by radio waves, these nuclei emit signals that are detected and converted into images.
    - **Tissue contrast**: MRI is exceptional at differentiating between soft tissues, such as the brain, muscles, tendons and ligaments.

- The MRI scanner
    - **Magnet**: Generates the powerful magnetic field required for the examination.
    - **Transmit/Receive Coils**: Transmit radio waves and detect the returned signals.
    - **The Examination Table: The** patient lies on this table, which moves inside the machine's tunnel.
    - **The Control Console**: Used by technologists to control the machine and observe images.

- Common Applications
    - **Neurology**: Detailed assessment of the brain and spinal cord.
    - **Orthopaedics**: Study of joints, ligaments and tendons.
    - **Cardiology**: Visualisation of the heart and blood vessels.
    - **Oncology**: detection and monitoring of tumours.
    - **Examination of internal organs**: such as the liver, kidneys and pelvic organs.

- Procedure
  - **Preparing the patient**: Removal of any metal objects, checking for metal implants or devices.
  - **Positioning**: The patient must remain still during the examination to ensure clear images.
  - **Contrast**: In some cases, a contrast agent may be used to improve visualisation.

- Benefits
  - **No X-rays**: MRI does not require ionising radiation, which makes it ideal for certain patients.
  - **Soft tissue accuracy**: Unrivalled ability to visualise and differentiate between the body's soft tissues.

- Disadvantages and concerns
  - **Duration**: MRI examinations may take longer than other imaging procedures.
  - **Claustrophobia**: The narrow MRI tunnel can be uncomfortable for some patients.
  - **Metal restrictions**: Metal objects or implants may be a contraindication or require special precautions.

- Technological developments
  - **Functional MRI (fMRI)**: Allows observation of brain activity by measuring variations in blood flow.
  - **Open-field MRI**: Designed to be less claustrophobic.
  - **Advanced imaging techniques**: Diffusion, perfusion and spectroscopy for more specialised studies.

MRI is a major advance in the world of medical imaging, offering doctors invaluable tools for diagnosing and treating a multitude of conditions. Its technical complexity is offset by its ability to provide images of exceptional clarity and precision, making this modality indispensable in modern medicine.

## • Ultrasonography

Ultrasonography, often referred to as ultrasound, is a medical imaging technique that uses high-frequency sound waves to produce images of the body's internal structures. It is commonly used to visualise foetuses during pregnancy, but its applications extend far beyond obstetrics.

- Fundamental principle
    - **Sound Wave Transmission**: A probe, called a transducer, emits sound waves that penetrate the body. These waves are reflected by internal structures.
    - **Echo and Image**: Reflected waves (echoes) are picked up by the transducer and transformed into an electronic image.

- Ultrasonography equipment
    - **The Transducer**: This is placed in direct contact with the patient's skin, often using a gel to facilitate wave transmission.
    - **The Console**: Where images are displayed and where the technologist can adjust various parameters to optimise the image.
    - **The Monitor**: Screen on which ultrasound images are displayed in real time.

- Common Applications
  - **Obstetrics**: Pregnancy monitoring and visualisation of the foetus.
  - **Cardiology**: Echocardiography to visualise the heart, its valves and blood flow.
  - **Abdominal organs**: Liver, kidneys, gall bladder, etc.
  - **Pelvic organs**: Uterus, ovaries, prostate.
  - **Vessel studies**: Doppler to assess blood flow.

- Procedure
  - **Patient preparation**: Depending on the area to be examined, specific instructions may be given, such as having a full bladder.
  - **Gel application**: A gel is applied to the area to be examined to ensure good conduction of the sound waves.
  - **Scanning with the transducer**: The technologist moves the transducer over the area of interest to obtain images.

- Benefits
  - **Non-invasive**: Ultrasound is a gentle procedure that generally requires no needles, dyes or radiation.
  - **Safety**: It is considered safe and is commonly used during pregnancy.
  - **Real-time**: Ultrasound offers real-time visualisation, ideal for visualising moving structures such as the heart.

- Limitations
  - **Interference with Air and Bone**: Sound waves do not penetrate well through air or bone, which can limit the visualisation of certain structures.

- **Image Quality**: Images can be affected by factors such as obesity or the presence of intestinal gas.

- Technological developments
  - **3D and 4D    ultrasound**: Allows structures to be viewed in three dimensions, and in "4D" (3D in motion).
  - **Elastography**: Evaluates tissue rigidity, useful in particular for assessing the degree of fibrosis in the liver.
  - **Enhanced    Contrast**: The use of special contrast agents to improve image quality in certain situations.

Ultrasonography is a versatile imaging modality with a wide range of medical applications. It is invaluable for its ability to provide images in real time without exposing the patient to radiation. Its non-invasive nature and relative simplicity make it an essential tool for many healthcare professionals.

## • Interventional imaging and other modalities

Interventional imaging encompasses imaging techniques that not only make it possible to visualise the inside of the body, but also to intervene to treat diseases or perform biopsies. It represents a bridge between diagnostic and therapeutic medicine. In addition to interventional imaging, there are other less common but equally important imaging modalities.

- Principle of Interventional Imaging
  - **Imaging guidance**: Using real-time images to guide medical instruments inside the body. The imaging techniques used often include X-rays, ultrasound and MRI.

- **Minimally invasive procedures**: In contrast to open surgery, interventional imaging often requires only small incisions or percutaneous entry points.

- Types of intervention
  - **Angioplasty and Stenting**: To open blocked arteries.
  - **Embolisation**: Blocking a blood vessel to prevent bleeding or treat a tumour.
  - **Radiofrequency ablation**: Destruction of tumours using heat.
  - **Biopsies:** Tissue samples taken for analysis.
  - **Drainage**: Removal of fluids or abscesses.

- Equipment and Technology
  - **Special X-ray tables**: Designed to support a variety of instruments and allow dynamic imaging.
  - **Catheters, Needles and Guide Wires**: Instruments used to navigate through the body.
  - **Contrast Agents**: To improve the visibility of blood vessels and organs.

- Advantages of Interventional Imaging
  - **Less invasive**: Reduces the risk of infection and recovery time.
  - **Alternative to Surgery**: Offers treatment options for patients who are not good candidates for surgery.
  - **Effectiveness**: Many of these procedures have comparable or even better success rates than traditional surgical techniques.

- Other Imaging Modalities
  - **Positron Emission Tomography (PET)**: Uses radioactive isotopes to detect areas of high

metabolic activity, often associated with tumours.
- **Mammography**: Specific breast imaging for the early detection of breast cancer.
- **Bone densitometry**: Measures bone mineral density to assess the risk of osteoporosis.
- **Fluoroscopic X-ray:** Provides real-time images of the inside of the body, often used to visualise the digestive system.

- Developments and the Future of Interventional Imaging
  - **Robotic interventions**: Using robotics for greater precision.
  - **Targeted therapies**: Direct administration of drugs or treatments to a specific area, minimising side effects.
  - **Imaging Fusion**: Combining different modalities to obtain complete and accurate images.

Interventional imaging and other imaging modalities play a crucial role in contemporary medicine. They offer innovative ways of diagnosing, treating and managing a variety of conditions, often reducing the need for more invasive procedures and improving patients' quality of life.

# Chapter 2:
# CAREGIVER'S DAILY NEWSPAPER IN RADIOLOGY

## The patient's arrival: preparation and welcome

Welcoming patients to a radiology department is one of the crucial stages in the diagnostic process. It is often the patient's first direct contact with the department, and its quality can influence the overall perception of the care received. Adequate preparation and a warm welcome are therefore essential to put patients at ease and ensure that examinations run smoothly.

- Making an appointment
  - **Preliminary information**: Briefly explain the procedure to the patient, mentioning any preparations (fasting, medication, etc.).
  - **Data collection**: medical history, allergies, possibility of pregnancy for women, etc.

- Welcome on arrival
  - **Reception and identification**: checking the patient's identity, confirming the appointment and the examination to be carried out.
  - **Soothing atmosphere**: Ensure that the reception area is clean, organised and reassuring for patients.

- Preparing the patient
  - **Cloakroom**: Provide clear instructions for changing clothes if necessary, and where to store personal belongings.

- **Health Questionnaire**: Fill in a detailed form on medical history, current medication, allergies, etc.
- **Explanation of the process**: Inform the patient of what to expect during the examination, how long it will take and what it may feel like.

- Expectation and comfort
    - **Waiting area**: Provide a comfortable space with magazines or distractions for waiting patients.
    - **Communication**: Regularly inform the patient of the remaining waiting time or any unforeseen delays.

- Informed Consent
    - **Information on the Review**: Explain the benefits, potential risks and alternatives.
    - **Signing the Consent**: Ensure that the patient has understood all the information provided and obtain his/her signature.

- Accompaniment to the examination room
    - **Guidance**: A member of staff should always accompany the patient to the examination room.
    - **Introduction to the team**: Briefly introduce the patient to the radiologist or technologist who will be carrying out the examination.

- After the exam
    - **Post-examination instructions**: Inform the patient of any potential side effects or precautions to be taken.
    - **Feedback**: Giving the patient the opportunity to ask questions or share concerns.

Welcoming and preparing patients is more than just an administrative procedure. They play a fundamental role in instilling confidence in the patient, in the efficiency of the examination and, ultimately, in the quality of care provided. A patient who is well informed and at ease is more likely to co-operate fully, which facilitates the work of the radiology team and optimises the accuracy of the results.

# Safety and protection against radiation

## • Basic principles of radiation protection

Radiation protection is an essential part of radiology and medical imaging practice. It aims to protect both patients and medical staff from the potentially harmful effects of ionising radiation. Several key principles guide this protection, ensuring that exposure is as low as reasonably achievable while providing quality diagnostic images.

- Justification
    - **Assessment of Risk vs. Benefit**: Any examination using radiation must be justified by weighing up the potential benefits for the patient against the risks associated with exposure.
    - **Alternatives**: Consider alternative non-radiation imaging modalities (such as MRI or ultrasound) if they can provide comparable diagnostic information.

- Optimisation
    - **Adapted settings**: Adjust the equipment settings according to the type of examination and the patient's morphology to minimise exposure.

- **Updating equipment**: Use modern, well-maintained machines that include dose reduction features.
- **Ongoing training**: Ensuring that staff are regularly trained in best practice and the latest developments in radiation protection.

- Limitation
  - **Exposure Limits**: Establish clear exposure limits for medical personnel to ensure their long-term safety.
  - **Personal monitoring**: Use of dosimeters to monitor personal exposure over time.

- Personal Protection
  - **Lead-coated clothing**: Use lead-coated aprons, goggles and gloves to protect against radiation during procedures or examinations.
  - **Protective screens**: Install screens or leaded walls to protect personnel during procedures.

- Information and Communication
  - **Information for patients**: Clearly explain the risks and benefits, and answer patients' questions about exposure.
  - **Standardised protocols**: Establish clear protocols for each type of examination to ensure a consistent and safe approach.

- Incident Management
  - **Emergency Protocols**: Have plans in place to respond to situations where there could be accidental overexposure.
  - **Analysis and feedback**: regular review of incidents to improve practices and prevent recurrence.

- Assessment and monitoring
  - **Regular Audits**: Carrying out regular checks on equipment and procedures to ensure that they comply with safety standards.
  - **Research and Development**: Keeping abreast of the latest research into radiation protection and adapting practices accordingly.

Radiation protection is a vital aspect of modern radiology. While recognising the incredible diagnostic and therapeutic benefits that medical imaging offers, it is essential to commit to protecting all those involved from the risk of unnecessary or excessive exposure.

## • Protection measures for staff

Staff working in medical imaging departments are potentially exposed to ionising radiation on a daily basis. In order to minimise the risks associated with this exposure, it is crucial to implement appropriate protective measures. These measures are designed to guarantee staff safety while enabling them to provide quality patient care.

- Personal Protective Equipment (PPE)
  - **Lead aprons**: These thick, heavy garments protect the body from exposure to radiation.
  - **Leaded gloves**: These protect the hands, which may be particularly close to the source of radiation during certain procedures.
  - **Leaded goggles**: These special goggles protect the eyes, which are sensitive to radiation.
  - **Thyroid shield:** A lead shield to protect the thyroid gland.

- Use of Dosimeters
  - **Constant monitoring**: Portable dosimeters record the amount of radiation to which a person is exposed.
  - **Regular analyses**: Dosimeter readings are checked periodically to ensure that exposure remains within safe limits.

- Protective Screens and Cabinets
  - **Sealed walls**: These barriers protect personnel from radiation when they are not directly involved in a procedure.
  - **Protected cabins**: Technologists can operate the machines from a radiation-proof cabin, protecting them from exposure.
- Distancing
  - **Distance principle**: The further away you are from a source of radiation, the less exposed you are. Staff are trained to keep as far away from the source as practicable.
  - **Use of long-handled tools**: To maintain a distance when handling near sources of radiation.

- Training and Education
  - **Regular sessions**: Staff receive ongoing training on best practice in radiation protection.
  - **Updates**: Keep up to **date** with the latest research and recommendations in the field of radiation protection.

- Protocols and Procedures
  - **Optimising examinations**: Carrying out examinations in such a way as to use the lowest possible radiation dose while obtaining quality images.

- **Checklists**: Use of checklists to ensure that all protection steps are followed.

- Equipment    Maintenance
  - **Regular        inspections**: Ensure that equipment is in good working order and does not present any additional risks.
  - **Upgrades**: Replacing older equipment with more modern, safer versions.

- Pregnancy Management
  - **Notification and follow-up**: Pregnant staff must declare their pregnancy so that additional measures can be taken to protect the foetus.
  - **Assignment to other tasks**: If possible, temporarily reposition pregnant workers to jobs with less or no exposure.

Protecting staff is a priority in any medical imaging department. By combining protective equipment, strict protocols, ongoing training and regular monitoring, it is possible to guarantee a safe working environment while providing high-quality patient care.

### • Patient protection

Patient safety is the cornerstone of any medical service, and radiology is no exception. When carrying out medical imaging examinations, it is imperative to protect patients from the potential risks associated with ionising radiation. Here's how it's done:

- Examination justification
  - **Risk-benefit assessment**: Before any radiological examination, it is crucial to ensure

that the potential benefits outweigh the risks associated with exposure to radiation.

- **Consultation**: The attending physicians, in collaboration with the radiologists, decide on the best examination for each patient.

- Optimising exposure
  - **Individual parameters**: The equipment is calibrated according to the patient's morphology, the area to be imaged and the clinical objective to minimise the dose while ensuring image quality.
  - **Standardised protocols**: The use of established protocols for common examinations ensures a minimum and uniform dose.

- Personal Protective Equipment for Patients
  - **Protective cushions and shields**: These devices, often leaded, are placed on or around the patient to protect organs that do not need to be exposed.
  - **Lead aprons for patients**: In some cases, a patient may wear a lead apron to protect certain parts of the body during the examination.

- Information and consent
  - **Preliminary discussion**: Before the examination, the patient is informed of the risks and benefits associated with the procedure.
  - **Informed Consent**: In certain situations, written consent is obtained to ensure that the patient understands and accepts the risks.

- Radiation-free alternatives
  - **Exploration of Other Options**: Where possible, non-radiation imaging techniques

such as ultrasound or MRI are considered as an alternative to X-ray or CT scan.

- Post-examination follow-up
  - **Monitoring**: In the rare event that an adverse reaction occurs, the patient is monitored and receives appropriate care.
  - **Exposure Register**: Some establishments keep a history of radiological exposures for each patient, making it possible to monitor cumulative exposure over time.

- Staff training
  - **Positioning techniques**: Staff are trained to position patients correctly to avoid unnecessary shots and to minimise exposure.
  - **Updates**: Staff receive regular training on new techniques and technologies to ensure patient safety.

- Maintaining and updating equipment
  - **Inspections**: The equipment is inspected regularly to ensure that it is operating correctly and safely.
  - **Investment**: Establishments are investing in modern technologies which often offer better quality images with lower doses.

Protecting patients is an ethical and professional commitment. By combining medical expertise, cutting-edge technology, ongoing training and transparent communication, we can ensure that every examination is both safe and effective.

# Effective communication
# with the medical team

Communication is an essential element in the medical field, particularly in medical imaging, where many specialities interact. Effective communication ensures optimal patient care, a better understanding of clinical needs and relevant, accurate test results. Here are the key aspects of effective communication with the medical team:

- Clarification of Examination Requests
    - **Precise wording**: Ensure that the examination request clearly states the type of examination required, the clinical reason and any relevant information about the patient.
    - **Discussion with the clinician**: In ambiguous cases, contact the attending physician to clarify the request and ensure that the examination is appropriate.

- Rapid Feedback
    - **Emergencies**: In urgent situations, rapidly transmit preliminary results to clinicians for immediate decision-making.
    - **Communication Platforms**: Use electronic communication systems, such as PACS (Picture Archiving and Communication Systems), to share images and reports.

- Multidisciplinary meetings
    - **Tumour Councils**: These meetings bring together specialists from various fields to discuss complex cancer cases.
    - **Case studies**: Present and discuss interesting or unusual cases with the team to enrich collective knowledge.

- Interdisciplinary Continuing Education
  - **Workshops**: Organise joint training sessions with other specialities to improve mutual understanding of roles and needs.
  - **Attending conferences**: Encourage the team to attend medical conferences to keep up to date with the latest advances and to network with other professionals.

- Constructive feedback
  - **Discussing techniques**: Discuss best practice and techniques for obtaining quality images with the team.
  - **Feedback on Reports**: Encourage clinicians to give feedback on radiology reports to improve the relevance and clarity of information.

- Ethics and Confidentiality
  - **Respect for privacy**: Ensuring that all communications concerning patients comply with confidentiality laws.
  - **Sensitive discussions**: Tactfully and professionally approach discussions about exam results, especially when the news is difficult.

- Managing Disparities of Opinion
  - **Open discussion**: If a member of the medical team disagrees with a result or interpretation, it is essential to open a respectful dialogue to understand the different perspectives.
  - **Expert consultation**: In complex cases, seek a second opinion or consult a specialist to clarify the situation.

Ultimately, effective communication with the medical team is the key to providing quality patient care. It fosters better collaboration, reinforces mutual trust and ensures that all the professionals involved have the information they need to make the best decisions for the patient.

# Understanding and anticipating the radiologist's needs

The role of the medical imaging orderly is crucial to the smooth running of the department. An important part of this role is to understand and anticipate the radiologist's needs. This leads to greater efficiency in diagnosis, reduced waiting times for patients and an overall improvement in patient care. Let's look at the key elements in responding effectively to the radiologist's needs.

- Mastery of imaging techniques
    - **Standardised protocols**: Know the standard procedures for each type of examination in order to prepare the patient correctly.
    - **Examination specifics**: Know how the different examinations differ in terms of preparation, positioning and duration.

- Adequate preparation of the patient
    - **Clinical history**: Gather essential information about the patient's state of health that may influence the interpretation of the images.
    - **Physical preparation**: Ensure that the patient is correctly positioned and comfortable to avoid artefacts and obtain clear images.

- Emergency Management
  - **Prioritisation**: Rapid identification of cases requiring immediate attention so that the radiologist can treat them as a priority.
  - **Communication**: Inform the radiologist of any relevant clinical information that could influence the urgency of the diagnosis.

- Organising and filing images
  - **Archiving systems**: Ensure that all images are correctly archived in systems, such as PACS, with relevant details to facilitate consultation by the radiologist.
  - **Annotations**: Add notes or markers to images where necessary to draw attention to areas of interest.

- Effective communication
  - **Transmission of information**: Provide the radiologist promptly with any additional information obtained during the examination or comments from the patient that may be relevant to the interpretation.
  - **Feedback**: Asking for feedback on image quality and adapting accordingly to meet the radiologist's needs for future examinations.

- Continuous updating of skills
  - **Training**: Regularly attend training courses to keep up to date with the latest techniques and technologies in medical imaging.
  - **Discussions with the radiologist**: Engage in discussions with the radiologist to better understand his or her needs and expectations.

- Optimised working environment
  - **Work area**: Ensure that the radiologist's work area is organised, clean and free from distractions.
  - **Equipment**: Ensure that all the necessary equipment, such as display screens, annotation tools or dictation systems, is working properly.

- Anticipating needs
  - **Timetable knowledge**: Know when the radiologist has busy periods or scheduled consultations to better manage patient flow.
  - **File preparation**: Gather in advance all files, previous images or other documents relevant to the planned cases.

By focusing on these elements, the carer can greatly facilitate the radiologist's work, improve the efficiency of the service and ensure that patients receive the best possible care. Close collaboration and open communication between the orderly and the radiologist are essential to achieving these goals.

# Chapter 3:
# TECHNIQUES AND
# SPECIFIC SKILLS

## Patient positioning
## for different procedures

Correct patient positioning during imaging procedures is essential to obtain accurate images and to ensure patient safety and comfort. Errors in positioning can lead to artefacts, non-diagnostic images or unnecessary radiation. Here is an overview of positioning for some of the most common imaging procedures:

- Chest X-ray
    - **Upright position**: Patient facing the detector plate, arms at his sides, shoulders relaxed and chin up.
    - **Lateral position**: Patient sideways, arms raised and hands clasped above the head.
- Abdominal X-ray
    - **Supine position**: The patient lies on his back with his arms at his sides.
    - **Lateral position (profile)**: Patient lying on his side, knees slightly bent.
- Radiography of the spine
    - **Antero-posterior (AP) position**: Patient facing the detector plate, arms raised.
    - **Lateral position**: Patient on his side, arms raised and legs slightly bent.

44

- Skull    X-ray
    - **Lateral position:** Patient's head turned to one side, ear pressed against the plate.
    - **AP position**: Patient facing the plate, mouth closed and Frankfurt plane parallel to the plate.
- Mammography
    - **Cranio-caudal        view (CC)**: The woman stands facing the machine, her breast is placed on the plate and gently compressed.
    - **Mediolateral    Oblique (MLO)**: The woman is positioned sideways, the breast is placed on the plate and compressed.
- Computer tomography (CT)
    - Positioning depends on the area to be examined. Generally, the patient lies on his or her back, with the arms either extended above the head or resting on the sides, depending on the area of the body being analysed.
- Magnetic Resonance Imaging (MRI)
    - As with CT, positioning depends on the area to be examined. Patients are often asked to cross their arms over their chest or leave them at their sides. Cushions or supports can be used to stabilise and comfort the patient.
- Ultrasonography
    - Positioning varies depending on the organ to be examined. For example, for a pelvic ultrasound, the patient might be supine with knees bent and feet in stirrups. For an abdominal ultrasound, the patient would be supine with the abdomen exposed.

It should be noted that precise positioning may vary depending on the equipment, clinical indications and the radiologist's preferences. The caregiver must always ensure that the patient is comfortable, safe and well-informed throughout the procedure. Clear communication is essential to reassure the patient and gain their co-operation.

# Help with administration contrast products

The use of contrast agents in medical imaging improves the visibility of certain structures or areas of the body. These agents are often necessary to obtain clear diagnostic images in modalities such as computer tomography (CT), magnetic resonance imaging (MRI) or radiography. Although nurses do not directly administer these products, they play a key role in the preparation, monitoring and management of patients. Here's a detailed exploration of that role.

- Understanding contrast media
  - **Nature and types**: Knowing how to distinguish between iodinated contrast agents (used in CT) and gadolinium-based agents (used in MRI), among others.
  - **How it works**: Find out how and why these agents improve the visibility of images.

- Prior assessment of the patient
  - **Medical history**: Identify any allergies, particularly to contrast products, and other possible contraindications (renal failure, for example).
  - **Informed consent**: Ensure that the patient understands the need for the contrast medium, its potential benefits and risks, and agrees to its administration.

- Preparing the patient
    - **Hydration**: Encourage patients to drink plenty of fluids before the examination, especially if iodinated contrast products are used.
    - **Fasting**: Depending on the protocols, inform patients if they need to fast before the procedure.
    - **Venous access**: Ensure that the patient has appropriate venous access, often a catheter, for administration of the product.

- Monitoring during administration
    - **Allergic reactions**: Monitor the patient carefully for signs of allergy or adverse reaction (rash, shortness of breath, dizziness, etc.).
    - **Patient comfort**: Some patients may feel a sensation of heat or a metallic taste during administration. Reassure them that this is normal.

- Post-administration care
    - **Post-examination hydration**: Encourage patients to drink plenty of water to help flush the contrast material from their system.
    - **Monitoring for side effects**: Although rare, side effects may occur after the examination. Inform patients of the symptoms to watch out for and when to consult a doctor.
    - **Removing the catheter**: If a catheter has been used, take care to remove it gently and disinfect the area.

- Communication with the medical team
    - **Sharing information**: Inform the radiologist or technician of any concerns about the patient, their condition or their reaction to the contrast medium.

- **Documentation**: Record all relevant information about the administration, including the type of agent used, the quantity, the time and any patient reaction.

- Training and updates
  - **Current knowledge**: As techniques and products evolve, it is crucial to keep abreast of the latest guidelines and recommendations concerning contrast agents.

The healthcare assistant plays a pivotal role in the patient experience during the administration of contrast media, ensuring both patient safety and the quality of the images obtained. Good training, effective communication and attention to the patient's needs are essential to fulfilling this role successfully.

# Post-examination follow-up: patient monitoring and comfort

After undergoing a medical imaging procedure, the patient may experience a variety of emotions and physical sensations. The post-examination phase is just as crucial as the procedure itself in ensuring the patient's safety, well-being and comfort. The nursing auxiliary has a fundamental role to play in this phase. Here is a detailed exploration of that role.

- Physical monitoring of the patient
  - **Vital signs**: Regularly check blood pressure, heart rate, respiration and temperature to ensure they remain within normal limits.
  - **Post-contrast reactions**: If a contrast agent has been administered, monitor for any allergic reactions or other adverse effects.

48

- **Post-interventional reactions**: If the patient has undergone an interventional procedure, watch for signs of bleeding, infection or other complications at the interventional site.

- Comfort assessment
  - **Pain or discomfort**: Ask the patient about any pain or discomfort experienced and take appropriate action.
  - **Positioning**: Make sure that the patient is comfortable, especially if he or she is going to be at rest for some time.

- Emotional support
  - **Anxiety and concerns**: Reassure patients, answer their questions and help them understand the next steps.
  - **Orientation**: Some examinations, particularly those under sedation, can be disorientating. Help them to come to their senses and understand their surroundings.

- Post-test instructions
  - **Medical instructions**: Provide clear instructions regarding medication, activities to be avoided and the possible need to return for follow-up.
  - **Hydration**: If a contrast agent has been used, remind the patient of the importance of drinking plenty of water to help eliminate it.

- Communication with the medical team
  - **Anomaly reports**: Inform the medical team immediately of any observations or concerns regarding the patient.
  - **Follow-up**: Know the follow-up process, including how and when the patient will receive

their results, and pass this information on to the patient.

- Patient discharge
  - **Discharge       process**: Ensure that the patient is stable and ready to leave the facility. Provide all necessary written and verbal instructions.
  - **Means of transport**: If the patient has been sedated or could be affected by the examination, ensure that they have a safe means of getting home.

- Documentation
  - **Follow-up notes**: Document all relevant details of post-examination follow-up, including the patient's condition, instructions given and any communication with the medical team.

Ensuring that patients feel cared for, safe and understood after the examination can have a significant impact on their overall experience of medical imaging. The caregiver's reassuring presence and constant attention are essential to ensure a smooth transition from the end of the examination to the patient's return to normal.

# Managing emergency situations in medical imaging

The medical imaging department is not immune to emergency situations. Whether it's a reaction to a contrast medium, sudden respiratory distress or a complication with a procedure, the orderly must be ready to respond quickly and effectively. Here is an in-depth approach to emergency management in medical imaging.

- Early    recognition of signs
    - **Monitoring**: Constant monitoring of vital signs can give early indications of an emerging problem.
    - **Observation**: Some patients may show subtle signs of discomfort or distress. Attention to detail, such as pallor, sweating or restlessness, can be crucial.

- Reaction to allergies
    - **Contrast agents**: Be aware of the signs of an allergic reaction to a contrast agent, such as skin rash, shortness of breath or swelling.
    - **Rapid intervention**: Have antihistamines or other emergency treatments available and know how to use them.

- Managing procedural    complications
    - **Bleeding**: How to stop bleeding, apply a dressing or prevent a haematoma.
    - **Infection**: Recognising the early signs of infection and how to manage them.

- Respiratory distress
    - **Airway obstruction**: Knowing how to clear a patient's airway, either manually or with a hoover.
    - **Resuscitation**: Have basic CPR skills (cardiopulmonary resuscitation) and know how to use an automatic defibrillator.

- Preparing for medical emergencies
    - **Emergency equipment**: Ensure that the department always has a well-stocked and up-to-date emergency trolley.
    - **Training**: Regular training in medical emergencies and simulations.

- Effective communication
  - **Alerting the team**: In an emergency, know who to call, whether it's the radiologist, the nursing staff or a resuscitation team.
  - **Patient information**: Reassure the patient while giving clear instructions on what to do (e.g. remain calm, breathe deeply).

- Post-emergency documentation
  - **Reports**: To document precisely what happened, the measures taken and the patient's condition after the emergency.
  - **Analysis and feedback**: After each emergency, organise debriefing meetings to assess what went well, what could have been done differently and how to improve preparedness in the future.

- Emotional support
  - **Patients**: Some patients may be traumatised by an emergency situation. Offer emotional support, listen to their concerns and reassure them.
  - **Yourself and colleagues**: Emergencies can also be stressful for staff. Encourage open discussion, mutual support and, if necessary, seek professional help to manage stress.

Medical imaging emergencies require rapid response, appropriate training and team coordination. The healthcare assistant, armed with the right skills and knowledge, can play a vital role in ensuring the safety and well-being of patients at these critical times.

# Chapter 4:
# ETHICS AND SENSITIVITY
# IN RADIOLOGY

## Respecting dignity and patient privacy

In the world of healthcare, where patients are often in vulnerable and exposed situations, respecting their dignity and privacy is not just a question of professionalism, it is a fundamental right of the patient. In medical imaging, where patients may have to undress or be positioned in a specific way for examinations, the importance of this consideration is accentuated. Here's a detailed approach to how the care assistant can ensure that the patient's dignity and privacy are respected.

- Transparent communication
    - **Explain the procedures**: Before starting, always tell the patient what is going to happen, why and how. This helps to reduce anxiety and uncertainty.
    - **Obtaining consent**: Before any examination or manipulation, make sure you obtain the patient's informed consent.

- Clothing management
    - **Suitable clothing**: Provide gowns or specific clothing that covers as much as possible, while allowing the necessary access for the examination.
    - **Private area**: Make sure the patient has a private area to change.

- Delicate positioning
    - **Respectful manoeuvres**: When positioning the patient, do so gently and respectfully. Explain each step to the patient and ask for their help whenever possible.
    - **Protecting intimate areas**: Use sheets or towels to cover areas that are not directly necessary for the examination.

- Cultural sensitivity
    - **Know the differences**: Some patients may have specific needs or concerns about intimacy because of their culture or religion. Be aware of these nuances and respect them.
    - **Staff preferences**: If a patient is more comfortable with a healthcare professional of the same sex, do your best to accommodate this, if possible.

- Confidentiality of information
    - **Data protection**: Patient information and test results must be treated with the utmost confidentiality. Discuss details only with the healthcare professionals concerned and in appropriate places.
    - **Image security**: Ensure that images or reports are stored securely and are only accessible to authorised persons.

- Managing delicate situations
    - **Anxious or embarrassed patients**: Offer reassurance, patience and empathy.
    - **Unexpected situations**: If a patient is suddenly emotional or upset, give them space, support and seek the help of a qualified healthcare professional if necessary.

- Continuing education
  - **Patient dignity education**: Take part in regular training courses focusing on respect for patient dignity and privacy to keep up to date with best practice and expectations.

Trust is a key element in the relationship between patient and healthcare professional. By scrupulously respecting the patient's dignity and privacy, the healthcare assistant creates an environment of trust that promotes not only the patient's well-being, but also the quality of the care provided.

# Understanding and managing patient anxiety

The experience of a medical imaging examination, although routine for healthcare professionals, can be a significant source of stress for many patients. Whether it's fear of the results, discomfort with the procedure or simply the unknown, patient anxiety can affect not only their overall experience, but also the quality of the images obtained. Here's how a caregiver can address and manage this anxiety.

- Recognition and empathy
  - **Active listening**: Ask open-ended questions to allow patients to express their concerns. A simple "How are you feeling today?" can open the door to a conversation.
  - **Empathetic responses**: Respond with compassion, showing that you understand their feelings. For example, "I can imagine how stressful this must be for you."

- Information and education
  - **Explain the procedure**: A lot of anxiety stems from fear of the unknown. Describing in detail what the patient can expect can alleviate some of these concerns.
  - **Time for questions**: Always leave space for the patient to ask questions and answer them honestly.

- A reassuring environment
  - **Room layout**: A well-lit, clean room with soothing elements (such as pictures or soft music) can help reduce anxiety.
  - **Professional attitude**: Your calm and assertiveness can have a calming effect on the patient.

- Relaxation techniques
  - **Deep breathing**: Encourage the patient to breathe deeply and slowly. This can help reduce tension and calm the mind.
  - **Distraction**: Talking about light subjects or offering headphones to listen to music can help distract patients from their nervousness.

- Advance preparation
  - **Written resources**: Providing brochures or leaflets describing the procedure can help patients to prepare themselves mentally in advance.
  - **Testimonials**: Sometimes listening to or reading about the experiences of other patients can reassure those who are anxious.

- Continuous presence
    - **Stay close by**: For some patients, knowing that a professional is nearby and ready to intervene can reduce anxiety.
    - **Constant feedback**: Keep the patient informed throughout the procedure about what is happening and what will happen next.

- Post-examination
    - **Debriefing**: After the procedure, take a few minutes to talk to the patient, answer any questions and reassure them.
    - **Tips for the next steps**: Let the patient know what's going to happen next, whether it's another examination, a follow-up appointment or waiting for the results.

The key to managing patient anxiety is communication, empathy and understanding. The carer, as the initial and constant point of contact for the patient, plays an essential role in creating a positive experience, despite the stress inherent in the medical examination.

# Informed consent in radiology

Informed consent is a crucial and ethical step in any medical intervention, ensuring that the patient is fully informed and in agreement with the proposed procedure. In radiology, this step is particularly relevant given the use of radiation, contrast media and other methods that may present risks to the patient. Here's a closer look at the concept and its application in radiology.

- Definition of informed consent
    - **A process, not just a document**: This is an ongoing communication between the

healthcare professional and the patient, not just the signing of a form.

- **Three key components**: Information, understanding and free will. The patient must receive all relevant information, understand it and make a decision without external pressure.

- The importance of radiology
    - **Radiation exposure**: Inform the patient of the potential risks associated with radiation exposure.
    - **Use of contrast agents**: Some patients may experience allergic reactions or other complications related to contrast agents.
    - **Invasive procedures**: Procedures such as image-guided biopsy require a clear understanding of the risks and benefits.

- Information to be provided
    - **Nature of the examination**: Detailed explanation of what the procedure involves.
    - **Expected benefits**: How the examination can help diagnose or treat a condition.
    - **Potential risks**: Side effects, complications or other possible consequences.
    - **Alternatives available**: Other examination or treatment options, if available.
    - What could happen if there is no examination: Consequences of not carrying out an examination.

- Implementation of the consent process
    - **Open discussion**: Leave enough time for an in-depth discussion with the patient.
    - **Simple language**: Avoid medical jargon and make sure the patient really understands.

- **Confirmation of understanding**: Encourage the patient to ask questions and rephrase what they have understood to check their understanding.
- **Documentation**: Provide an informed consent form for you to sign, but make sure this follows a thorough discussion.

- Special considerations
  - **Minors and guardians**: In the case of minor patients, consent must be obtained from the parents or legal guardians.
  - **Patients unable to give consent**: For patients who are unable to understand or communicate, alternative means of obtaining informed consent should be sought, such as through a legal representative.
  - **Emergency situations**: In time-critical situations, informed consent may be modified, but the importance of information should not be minimised.

- Refusal and withdrawal of consent
  - **Right to refuse**: Patients always have the right to refuse a procedure, even after giving their consent.
  - **Managing refusal**: Listen to the patient's concerns, provide additional information if necessary, but always respect their decision.

Informed consent in radiology is not only an ethical and legal obligation, it also guarantees patient trust and collaboration. By understanding and respecting their rights, healthcare professionals can ensure patient-centred care and optimal outcomes.

# Navigate in common ethical dilemmas

Radiology, like all medical fields, is faced with complex ethical dilemmas that can influence clinical decision-making and the relationship between patient and healthcare professional. For a healthcare assistant working in radiology, understanding these dilemmas and knowing how to approach them is essential. Here is an exploration of some of these common ethical dilemmas and how to deal with them.

- Conflicts between clinical benefit and patient risk
    - **Context**: Although exposure to radiation is often necessary for a precise diagnosis, it does present risks. Where do we draw the line between benefit and risk?
    - **Navigation**: The patient's need for diagnosis and treatment must be balanced with the need to minimise radiation exposure. An open discussion with the radiologist and the patient is essential.

- Informed consent versus imperative need for diagnosis
    - **Context**: What should be done if a patient refuses a necessary examination for personal reasons, despite the potential risks to their health?
    - **Navigation**: Listen to the patient's concerns, offer alternatives if possible and respect their autonomy while emphasising the medical importance of the examination.

- Confidentiality and right to information
    - **Context**: Who should have access to radiological images and reports? How should requests from family or other professionals be managed?

- **Navigation**: Make sure you are aware of the laws on the confidentiality of medical data in your country and always respect the patient's right to confidentiality.

- Error management
  - **Context**: What happens if you identify a potential error in a report or image? Or if you realise that the wrong patient has been examined?
  - **Navigation**: Honesty and transparency are essential. Inform the radiologist immediately and consider informing the patient according to the protocols in place.

- Inequalities in access to healthcare
  - **Context**: Not all patients have the same access to advanced imaging techniques. How can this imbalance be managed?
  - **Navigation**: Do your best to treat all patients fairly and advocate for equitable resources and services where possible.

- Economic     pressures
  - **Context**: The pressure to speed up examinations and increase throughput can affect the quality of care.
  - **Navigation**: The priority must always be the patient's safety and well-being. If you feel pressure that could compromise the quality of care, discuss it with management or consider other channels of communication.

- Technological advances versus ethics
  - **Context**: New technologies can provide more detailed images, but at what cost? And when do machines replace human judgement?

- **Navigation**: Keep up to date with technological advances and their ethical implications. Human clinical judgement will always be essential.

Navigating ethical dilemmas requires a deep understanding of ethical principles, open communication and a commitment to the well-being of the patient. It is essential that carers, in collaboration with the whole radiology team, actively reflect on ethical issues and seek training and resources to address these issues in an informed way.

# Chapter 5:
# DEVELOPMENTS AND PROFESSIONAL OPPORTUNITIES

## Continuing education and possible specialisations

Radiology is a constantly evolving field, with rapid technological advances and the emergence of new methodologies and techniques. For a healthcare assistant working in radiology, it's essential to stay up to date and consider specialisations to improve your skills and provide the best possible patient care. Here is an overview of the continuing education and specialisation options available to a radiology orderly.

- Importance of continuing training
    - **Adapting to technological advances**: radiology equipment is constantly being improved, offering better quality images and new functions.
    - **Improved patient care**: Continuing training enables you to improve your skills in patient care, particularly for complex or rare cases.
    - **Career development**: This opens the door to more specialised positions or greater responsibilities.

- Types of continuing training
    - **Workshops and seminars**: These short courses often focus on specific subjects and offer immersion in new techniques or case studies.

- **Online courses**: Many institutions offer online learning modules tailored to radiology professionals.
- **Degree courses**: For those who wish to deepen their knowledge, there are degree programmes that can be spread over several months or years.

- Possible specialisations
  - **Paediatric radiology**: Focus on imaging children, which requires special precautions and specific training.
  - **Interventional radiology**: This sub-specialty combines imaging and the performance of minimally invasive medical procedures.
  - **Management and administration in radiology**: For those wishing to manage a radiology team or department.
  - **Radiation protection**: Specialising in techniques and methods for guaranteeing the safety of patients and staff in the face of radiation.
  - **Training and teaching**: Passing on your knowledge to the next generation of care assistants and other radiology professionals.

- How do I choose a specialism?
  - **Identify your interests**: What aspects of the job do you want to focus on? What are you most passionate about?
  - **Evaluate career opportunities**: Certain specialisations may offer better employment or progression opportunities.
  - **Consider the duration and cost of the training**: Some programmes may be more accessible than others, both in terms of cost and duration.

- Keeping up to date
  - **Membership of professional associations**: These organisations often offer resources, training and networking opportunities for their members.
  - **Attending conferences**: Attending radiology conferences can provide an insight into the latest advances and trends in the field.
  - **Professional reading**: Newspapers, magazines and specialist books can help you keep abreast of the latest research and innovations.

Continuing education and specialisation are not only ways of improving your skills, but also of providing better patient care and developing your career. For a radiology orderly, investment in learning and professional growth is essential for a fulfilling and impactful career.

# The radiology of the future: what is the role of the care assistant?

As the 21st century advances, radiology is undergoing radical transformation thanks to technology, automation and artificial intelligence. These changes will influence the role of all professionals working in medical imaging, including healthcare assistants. Let's take a look at the future of radiology and what it means for the nursing auxiliary.

- Increasing integration of Artificial Intelligence (AI)
  - **Automation of routine tasks**: With AI analysing images, many basic tasks can be automated, freeing up time for professionals.

- **The carer's role**: to monitor and interact with these AI systems, to ensure the quality of images before they are analysed and to familiarise themselves with alerts or notifications.

- More advanced imaging modalities
  - **Emergence of new techniques**: New modalities or improved versions of existing techniques will continue to emerge.
  - **Role of the care assistant**: To be trained to assist in these new techniques, to understand their advantages and limitations, and to explain these procedures to patients.

- Patient-centred care
  - **Improved communication thanks to technology**: Integrated systems will enable better communication between medical teams.
  - **The carer's role**: to use these systems to ensure a smooth flow of information and to play an active part in coordinating the patient's care.

- Virtual imaging environments
  - **Simulations and augmented reality**: These technologies could be used for training or even to guide certain interventions.
  - **Role of the nursing auxiliary**: Taking part in these virtual training sessions, assisting radiologists during procedures assisted by augmented reality.

- Teleradiology and remote care
  - **Expansion of remote services**: With telemedicine on the rise, radiology is no exception.

- **Role of the healthcare assistant**: Assisting patients during teleradiology sessions, ensuring that the equipment is working properly, and facilitating remote communication.

- Training and education
  - **New learning methods**: Virtual and augmented reality, as well as other technological tools, will transform radiology training.
  - **The role of the nursing auxiliary**: Keeping up to date with these new learning methods, taking an active part in continuing training.

- Ethical and regulatory issues
  - **Navigating a changing landscape**: With the emergence of new technologies, new ethical and regulatory issues will arise.
  - **The role of the care assistant**: Being aware of ethical dilemmas, taking part in training on new regulations, and ensuring that care is always patient-centred.

The radiology of the future promises to be both exciting and complex. Although technology will play a predominant role, the importance of the human element - compassion, empathy, communication - will remain central. The healthcare assistant, as the essential link between technology and the patient, will continue to play a crucial role in providing high-quality care in the ever-evolving field of radiology.

# Networking and professional development

Professional development is not just about acquiring new technical skills or pursuing formal studies. Networking, i.e. the creation and maintenance of professional relationships, is a crucial aspect of career advancement, discovering opportunities and enriching knowledge. In the world of radiology, this is all the more true given the rapid pace of technological and clinical change.

- Why is networking crucial?
    - **Access to opportunities**: Many jobs and training opportunities are never advertised, but are instead passed on by word of mouth.
    - **Sharing knowledge**: Meetings with peers provide an opportunity to exchange information, techniques and case studies.
    - **Mentoring**: Strong professional relationships can lead to mentoring relationships, which are invaluable for professional growth.
    - **Collaboration**: Established relationships can lead to collaboration on projects, research or other initiatives.

- Where and how to network?
    - **Conferences and seminars**: These events attract professionals from a variety of backgrounds and often offer dedicated networking opportunities.
    - **Professional associations**: Many radiology-related associations organise events, workshops and meetings for their members.
    - **Professional social networks**: Sites like LinkedIn can be used to establish and maintain professional relationships.

- **Training courses and workshops**: Taking part in training courses can put you in contact with trainers and other participants with similar interests.
- **Hospitals and clinics**: Take an active part in events or internal groups dedicated to radiology or medicine.

- Tips for effective networking
    - **Be authentic**: It's not just about taking, but also about giving. Share your knowledge and be willing to help others.
    - **Prepare a short introduction**: Knowing how to introduce yourself briefly and effectively is essential when meeting people.
    - **Stay up to date**: Keep abreast of the latest developments in radiology so you can discuss relevant topics.
    - **Follow up**: After meeting someone, send a message or email to thank them and express your interest in staying in touch.
    - **Stay active**: Networking is an ongoing effort. Try to regularly attend events or participate in online discussions.

- Professional development    management
    - **Plan ahead**: Set professional goals and identify how networking can help you achieve them.
    - **Stay organised**: Keep track of the people you meet, upcoming events and opportunities to explore.
    - **Ask for feedback**: Sometimes an outside perspective can offer valuable insights into your career or skills.

Networking, when approached proactively and thoughtfully, can be a major asset to the professional development of anyone working in radiology. By investing time and effort in building meaningful relationships, healthcare assistants can not only broaden their professional horizons, but also make a significant contribution to the radiology community as a whole.

# Chapter 6:
# TESTIMONIALS AND EXPERIENCES

## Typical and atypical days:
## stories from care assistants

Radiology, like many other medical fields, offers a variety of experiences. Every day brings its share of learning experiences, challenges and surprises. Through the stories of care assistants, we delve into the day-to-day realities and exceptional situations of this profession.

### A typical day
* *Julie, care assistant for 5 years*

Julie usually starts her day by checking the appointment schedule. After preparing the examination rooms, she welcomes the first patients. Most of her time is spent preparing patients for their examinations, ensuring their comfort and working with the radiology technician. Communication is essential: explaining procedures, reassuring anxious patients and ensuring that patients are positioned correctly. The end of the day is often spent disinfecting rooms, putting equipment away and preparing for the next day.

### An unusual day
* *Antoine, care assistant in the radiology department for 3 years*

Antoine remembers one day when the main X-ray equipment broke down. While managing the patients already present, the team had to quickly reorganise the day, sending some patients home and prioritising urgent cases using the secondary equipment. At the same time, an anxious patient had an allergic reaction to a contrast agent. Antoine had to manage the situation in collaboration with the medical team, while reassuring the other patients in the waiting room.

### An exceptional day
- *Sofia, care assistant for 8 years*

Sofia recounts a day marked by the unexpected arrival of a celebrity on the ward. While keeping her identity confidential, the team had to manage the excitement that this created. It was a balancing act between providing quality care, respecting the privacy of the celebrity and managing the curiosity of other patients and staff.

### A rewarding day
- *Kévin, care assistant in radiology for 2 years*

Kévin talks about a day when he looked after a non-French-speaking patient with a hearing impairment. Thanks to his sign language skills, which he had learnt during further training, he was able to communicate with the patient, put him at ease and ensure a smooth procedure. That day, he felt a great sense of professional satisfaction, having been able to make a difference for this patient.

These stories highlight the variability of experiences in radiology. They show that while every day may seem typical on the surface, there is never a shortage of challenges, surprises and learning opportunities for radiology orderlies.

# The challenges and rewards of the job

Being a radiology orderly, like other medical professions, is full of challenges and rewards. Although each day can present its own obstacles, the rewards and achievements provide the gratification that motivates many professionals to pursue their careers with passion.

Challenges
- **Workload and stress**: The growing demand for medical imaging services often means busy days. Managing a busy schedule while ensuring that every patient receives quality care can be stressful.
- **Technological updating**: Rapidly evolving imaging technologies require ongoing training to keep up to date, which can be difficult to reconcile with day-to-day work.
- **Managing anxious patients**: Anxiety surrounding medical procedures is common, and it can be difficult to reassure and calm some patients.
- **Health risks**: Despite radiation protection measures, radiology professionals are potentially exposed to radiation. They must therefore always be vigilant.
- **Emotional issues**: Healthcare assistants may encounter patients in complex or distressing medical situations, which can have an emotional impact.

Awards
- **Positive impact on patient health**: Playing a central role in the diagnosis and treatment of patients is extremely rewarding. A good diagnosis can change a patient's life.
- **Continuous professional development**: The need to keep up to date with technology offers numerous opportunities for training and career development.
- **Relationships with patients**: Many care assistants enjoy day-to-day interactions with patients and find it rewarding to offer support and reassurance.
- **Professional recognition**: Working in a specialised field such as radiology offers a degree of recognition.

The skills and expertise of care assistants are valued by other health professionals.
- **Everyday variety**: No day in radiology is the same. The different cases, procedures and challenges make each day unique.
- **Satisfaction of working in a team**: Radiology is teamwork. Working with radiologists, technicians and other professionals gives you a sense of belonging and camaraderie.

Ultimately, despite the challenges inherent in being a radiology orderly, the many rewards, both professional and personal, make the profession deeply rewarding.

# Advice for novices and students

The transition from theoretical training to clinical practice can be a monumental leap for many radiology students and novices. Here are a few tips to ease the transition and ensure a rewarding experience right from the start.
- **Cultivate your curiosity**: Radiology technology and protocols are constantly evolving. Maintain an attitude of constant learning, ask questions and don't be afraid to admit what you don't know.
- **Build solid professional relationships**: Your team is your greatest resource. Get to know your colleagues, exchange experiences and seek advice. Teamwork is fundamental in radiology.
- **Practise empathic communication**: Your interactions with patients will vary. Some may be anxious or frightened. Active listening and empathy can help to establish a relationship of trust.
- **Be patient**: Your training has given you the basics, but mastery comes with practice. Expect to make mistakes, but see them as learning opportunities.

- **Think about your safety**: Familiarise yourself with the radiation protection protocols and follow them scrupulously. Safety must always be a priority, both for you and for your patients.
- **Keep a balance between your professional and personal life**: Being a radiology orderly can be a demanding job. Make sure you take time for yourself, rest and recharge.
- **Take advantage of continuing education opportunities**: The field of radiology offers many specialisations and technological advances. Take part in seminars, workshops and other training courses to broaden your skills.
- **Stay organised**: Good time management and organisation can help manage your workload and reduce stress. Find a system that works for you and stick to it.
- **Seek mentoring**: If possible, find an experienced mentor who can guide you, give you practical advice and help you navigate the early stages of your career.
- **Keep up to date**: Subscribe to professional journals, take part in online forums or discussion groups to keep abreast of the latest news and trends in the field.
- **Prepare for difficult days**: Not every day will be perfect. There will be challenges, surprises and stressful moments. Have a strategy for dealing with these moments, whether it's talking to a trusted colleague, practising meditation or writing in a journal.
- **Celebrate your successes**: Even small victories, such as a particularly grateful patient or a technique mastered, deserve to be celebrated. Take the time to acknowledge your successes and those of your team.

Stepping into the world of radiology as a novice can be daunting, but with the right support, preparation and attitude, it can also be extremely rewarding. Embrace every experience as an opportunity to learn and grow in your career.

# Chapter 7:
# HARDWARE AND TECHNOLOGY IN RADIOLOGY

## Understanding how it works

### • Maintenance and cleaning

The maintenance and cleaning of radiology equipment are essential to ensure that it operates at optimum efficiency and to guarantee the safety and well-being of patients and staff. These tasks require special attention because they have a direct impact on the quality of the images produced and the overall efficiency of the department.

1. Importance of maintenance and cleaning
   - **Equipment reliability**: Well-maintained equipment is less likely to break down, reducing downtime and associated costs.
   - **Image quality**: Clean, well-maintained machines produce better quality images, which are essential for accurate diagnosis.
   - **Patient and staff safety**: Maintenance reduces the risk of accidental exposure to radiation and ensures that protective devices are working properly. In addition, clean equipment minimises the risk of nosocomial infections.

2. Maintenance procedures
   - **Preventive maintenance**: This involves regular inspections and servicing of equipment to prevent potential breakdowns. This includes calibration, software updates, replacement of worn parts and performance testing.

- **Corrective maintenance**: This is carried out in response to a fault or breakdown. The aim is to repair or replace defective parts of the equipment.

3. Cleaning protocols
   - **Daily cleaning**: Remove dust and debris with soft cloths. Frequent contact surfaces, such as knobs and handles, should be cleaned with mild disinfectants to prevent the spread of germs.
   - **Thorough cleaning**: Depending on the frequency of use and the manufacturer's recommendations, a more thorough cleaning should be carried out. This may include the use of specific disinfectant solutions and partial dismantling of the equipment for a thorough cleaning.
   - **Cleaning after contamination**: In the event of contact with body fluids or other contaminants, immediate cleaning and disinfection are essential.

4. Training and awareness-raising
   - Staff using the equipment must be trained in the appropriate cleaning and maintenance protocols. This ensures that everyone is on the same wavelength and complies with standards.
   - It is also essential to be aware of the signs that equipment requires maintenance, such as changes in image quality, unusual noises or recurring malfunctions.

5. Documentation and follow-up
   - All maintenance and cleaning operations must be logged. This ensures proper monitoring and helps identify trends or recurring problems.

Ultimately, maintenance and cleaning in radiology is about more than keeping equipment in good condition. It's about ensuring that every patient receives the highest quality care in a safe and hygienic environment.

## • Recent and future innovations

Radiology, like many medical fields, is constantly evolving thanks to technological advances and scientific discoveries. Here's a look at recent innovations and future trends that could shape the medical imaging landscape in the years to come.

1. Recent innovations
   - **Artificial intelligence (AI) and machine learning**: These technologies help radiologists to analyse images faster and more accurately. Algorithms can detect anomalies that the human eye might miss.
   - **Digital radiology**: Less radiation is needed to produce high-quality images, reducing exposure for patients.
   - **Hybrid imaging**: Technologies such as PET-MRI combine imaging modalities to provide a more complete picture of the human body.
   - **3D and 4D imaging**: These techniques offer a more detailed and dynamic view of internal structures, which is particularly useful in obstetrics and cardiology.

2. Expected innovations
   - **Augmented radiology**: The use of augmented reality could help radiologists to superimpose radiological images on the patient's body in real time during procedures.
   - **Automation**: As AI develops, many processes could be automated, including making appointments, triaging cases according to urgency and even the initial analysis of images.
   - **Portable technologies**: Like portable ultrasound scanners, other imaging devices could become more compact, allowing doctors to take their equipment with them.

- **Molecular imaging**: This technology goes beyond the visualisation of structures to show what is happening at a molecular level, offering valuable information about diseases and their progression.
- **Distance learning and teleradiology**: With advances in communications technology, it is likely that more and more training and diagnosis will be carried out remotely, enabling radiologists to work and learn from anywhere.
- **Predictive imaging**: Thanks to AI and in-depth data analysis, it could be possible to predict the progression of a disease or a patient's susceptibility to certain conditions on the basis of their images.

3. Challenges and considerations

While offering great promise, these innovations also come with challenges. The protection of patient data, the need for ongoing training for healthcare professionals, and the high cost of some new technologies are major concerns. In addition, it is crucial to ensure that these innovations increase precision and efficiency without compromising the quality of care.

Radiology is at the forefront of many exciting advances in medicine, and the coming years promise to be full of discoveries and innovations that will continue to transform the field.

# Accessories and additional equipment

## • Examination tables, covers and cushions

In a radiology department, patient comfort and safety are paramount. Examination tables, covers and cushions play an essential role in this respect. These elements guarantee not only the patient's well-being but also the quality of the images obtained.

1. Examination tables
- **Ergonomic design**: Modern and designed for maximum comfort, the examination tables are height-adjustable and can be tilted or moved in different directions to suit different types of radiological examination.
- **Load capacity**: The tables are designed to support patients of different weights, with capacities of up to 200 kg or more, depending on the model.
- **Technological integration**: Many tables are equipped with integrated sensors and other technologies that interact directly with the radiology equipment, facilitating image acquisition.

2. Table covers
- **Protection against infection**: Disposable covers are used to minimise the risk of spreading infection. They are removed and replaced after each patient.
- **Increased comfort**: Some covers are padded or made from soft materials to improve patient comfort during the examination.
- **Ease of use**: They are often designed to be easily removable and disposable, guaranteeing optimum hygiene with minimal effort.

3. Cushions and supports
- **Precise positioning**: Cushions are essential for positioning the patient precisely, ensuring the best possible image quality. They can be placed under the head, neck, knees or other parts of the body.
- **Movement reduction**: The cushions also help to stabilise the patient, reducing involuntary movements that could compromise image quality.

- **Radiolucent materials**: These cushions are often made from special materials that do not interfere with radiation, ensuring that they do not appear on X-ray images.
- **Hygiene and cleanability**: As with examination tables, it is crucial that cushions and supports are easy to clean and disinfect.

Examination tables, covers and cushions play a discreet but crucial role in radiology. They ensure patient comfort while guaranteeing image quality. As technology evolves, we can expect to see new innovations in this equipment, combining functionality, safety and comfort even more effectively.

## • Restraint systems and positioning aids

Restraints and positioning aids are essential to ensure that the patient remains stable and in the correct position during radiology procedures. This not only helps to obtain high-quality images, but also ensures patient safety and comfort. Here is a detailed explanation of these devices and their importance.

1. Why use restraints and positioning aids?
- **Reduce movement**: Any movement, however slight, can cause an image to become blurred or less clear, making diagnosis more difficult.
- **Ensuring comfort**: Positioning a patient correctly can reduce discomfort, especially during prolonged examinations.
- **Protecting the patient**: In some procedures, it is essential that the patient remains in a specific position to avoid injury.

## 2. Types of restraint

- **Velcro straps**: These adjustable straps can be used to gently hold the patient's limbs in place.
- **Splints:** Mainly used to immobilise a specific part of the body, such as the arm or leg.
- **Harnesses and belts**: Can be used to stabilise the patient's trunk.

## 3. Positioning aids

- **Wedges and foam blocks**: These devices, often radiolucent, help to elevate or support a part of the body to obtain the desired angle for imaging.
- **Inflatable cushions**: These can be adjusted to provide the right level of support where needed.
- **Positioning straps**: These can be used to hold the patient in a specific position, such as during a spinal examination.
- **Positioning plates**: These rigid plates can be placed under the patient to provide stable support.

## 4. Considerations when using restraint devices and positioning aids

- **Communication**: It is essential to explain to the patient why the device is needed and to ensure that they are comfortable throughout the procedure.
- **Regular checking**: Staff should check regularly to ensure that the device is not too tight or uncomfortable.
- **Training**: Staff must be properly trained on how and when to use these devices, based on best practice and safety protocols.

Restraints and positioning aids play a crucial role in radiology, ensuring that images are clear and accurate, while keeping the patient safe and comfortable. By using these tools correctly, radiology professionals can provide quality care while ensuring the well-being of their patients.

# The importance of collaboration with radiology technicians

The world of radiology is complex and multidisciplinary, requiring the close collaboration of different professionals to function effectively. One of the most crucial partnerships is that between the care assistant and the radiology technician. The complementary nature of their roles is essential to guarantee the quality of care, patient safety and efficiency of the service. Let's take a closer look at the importance of this collaboration.

1. Expertise and complementary skills
   - **Role of the radiology technician**: They are specifically trained to handle radiology equipment, interpret medical prescriptions and carry out examinations under the required technical conditions.
   - **Role of the healthcare assistant**: They support patients throughout the process, ensuring their comfort and safety and making sure they are correctly positioned for the examination.

2. Improving the quality of care
   - **Preparing the patient**: The healthcare assistant plays a crucial role in preparing the patient for the examination, ensuring that all metal objects are removed, explaining the procedure and reassuring anxious patients.
   - **Precise positioning**: By working together, the technician and assistant ensure that the patient is correctly positioned, which is vital for obtaining high-quality images.

3. Increased service efficiency
   - **Optimised workflow**: Good communication between care assistants and technicians ensures that patients are ready and positioned on time, avoiding delays.

- **Discussing specific needs**: If a patient requires special care or has specific needs, the care assistant can inform the technician beforehand.

4. Patient safety
- **Continuous monitoring**: While the technician concentrates on the machine and obtaining clear images, the carer can monitor the patient's well-being, making sure they are not experiencing any pain or discomfort.
- **Emergency interventions**: In the event of a problem, such as an allergic reaction to the contrast medium, rapid and effective collaboration between the care assistant and the technician is essential.

5. Professional development
- **Mutual learning**: By working side by side, orderlies and technicians can learn from each other, broadening their respective understanding of the different aspects of radiology.
- **Feedback**: A technician can provide valuable feedback to the care assistant on how to improve patient positioning or preparation, and vice versa.

The collaboration between nursing assistants and radiology technicians is more than the sum of its parts. Together, they ensure that the radiology department runs smoothly, that patients receive high-quality care, and that the images produced are accurate and informative. This symbiosis is essential to the success of any radiology department.

# Chapter 8:
# HEALTH AND WELLBEING
# OF THE ORDERLY

## Recognising and preventing burnout

Burnout is a complex syndrome that can affect anyone, especially healthcare professionals. For those working in radiology, the specific challenges of the job, constant pressure and long hours can lead to this phenomenon. It is essential to recognise the early signs and take preventive measures to ensure the well-being of staff.

1. Understanding burnout
   - **Definition**: Burnout is characterised by emotional exhaustion, depersonalisation (a feeling of detachment from patients or work) and a reduced sense of personal accomplishment.
   - **Risk factors in radiology**: High workload, pressure to minimise errors, constantly evolving technology requiring continuous training, demanding patient-caregiver interactions, and possible isolation in dark areas without direct contact with other colleagues.

2. Signs and symptoms
   - **Emotional**: Feelings of emptiness, loss of empathy, irritability, isolation and increased sensitivity to criticism.
   - **Physical**: Chronic fatigue, sleep disorders, headaches or muscle pain, and reduced immunity.
   - **Behavioural**: Procrastination, neglect of tasks, lateness or absence from work, and social isolation.
   - **Cognitive**: Difficulty concentrating, frequent forgetfulness and impulsive decisions.

3. Preventive measures
- **Work-life balance**: It's crucial to have time for yourself, to relax and engage in activities outside work.
- **Regular breaks**: Take short but frequent breaks during the day to relax and get away from the work environment.
- **Social support**: Maintaining strong relationships with colleagues and seeking support when you feel overwhelmed.
- **Training and mentoring**: Having access to ongoing training and mentoring opportunities can help you feel more competent and less isolated.
- **Time management and delegation**: Learn how to manage your time effectively and delegate tasks where possible.

4. Institutional support
- **Raising awareness among management**: Establishments must recognise the importance of staff well-being and put measures in place to reduce the risk of burnout.
- **Wellness programmes**: offering resources such as counselling, stress management workshops and relaxation areas.
- **Regular feedback**: Organise regular meetings with staff to discuss their concerns and adjust the workload if necessary.

5. Seeking help
- If a professional suspects the onset of burnout, it is crucial to consult a mental health professional. Recognising the problem early and seeking help can prevent more serious consequences.

Burnout in radiology can have serious consequences, not only for the professional themselves, but also for the quality of care provided to patients. Recognising the early signs and taking preventive action is essential to ensure the well-being and mental health of radiology professionals.

## The importance of physical health: preventing musculoskeletal injuries

Radiology professionals, including orderlies and technicians, often spend long hours in non-ergonomic postures, moving heavy equipment or helping to position patients. This exposes them to an increased risk of musculoskeletal injuries. Preventing these injuries is crucial to ensuring the well-being of staff and the continuity of patient care.

1. Understanding musculoskeletal injuries
   - **Definition**: Injuries that affect the musculoskeletal system, including muscles, tendons, ligaments, nerves, discs and blood vessels.
   - **Common causes in radiology**: Repetitive movements, inappropriate lifting, prolonged posture, overhead work and inappropriate patient handling.

2. Risk identification
   - **Heavy equipment**: Healthcare assistants and technicians frequently move equipment, such as examination tables or restraining devices.
   - **Patient positioning**: Helping patients to get on or off the table, or to position themselves correctly for an examination, can place strain on the back and limbs.
   - **Prolonged postures**: Standing for long periods, especially if your posture is inadequate, can cause pain and injury.

3. Preventive measures
- **Ergonomic training**: Providing training in ergonomic principles, teaching staff how to work efficiently while protecting their health.
- **Mechanical aids**: Using assistive devices to lift and move patients or equipment, thereby reducing the physical burden on staff.
- **Workplace layout**: Ensure that equipment is at an appropriate height, minimising the need to bend or stretch.
- **Breaks and stretching**: Encourage regular breaks and the adoption of stretching routines to avoid muscle tension.

4. Raising awareness and a culture of prevention
- **Management support**: It is crucial that management understands the importance of preventing musculoskeletal injuries and provides the necessary resources.
- **Regular feedback**: Enable staff to report potential problems and encourage open communication about risks.

5. Rapid intervention
- If an injury does occur, early intervention is crucial. Early re-education and rehabilitation can prevent a minor injury from becoming chronic.

The physical health of radiology professionals is crucial, not only to their personal well-being, but also to ensuring quality patient care. The recognition and prevention of musculoskeletal injuries must be a priority for all healthcare establishments. By investing in training, equipment and a culture of prevention, the risk of these injuries can be greatly reduced.

# Mental health in a medical environment

The mental health of healthcare professionals is an essential element in guaranteeing quality patient care. The medical environment, with its constant challenges, emergencies and stress, can have a significant impact on the emotional well-being of staff. It is therefore vital to understand the specific challenges associated with mental health in this context and to put in place appropriate support measures.

1. Recognising the unique challenges of the medical environment
  - **Emotional burden**: Healthcare professionals are regularly confronted with illness, suffering and, sometimes, death. This can lead to feelings of sadness, guilt or powerlessness.
  - **Workload and irregular hours**: Long hours, night shifts and constant urgency can contribute to burnout and other mental health problems.
  - **Difficult interactions**: Whether with patients, families or even colleagues, tensions and conflicts can arise, creating additional stress.

2. Signs of mental health problems
  - Social withdrawal, irritability or mood swings.
  - Reduced professional performance.
  - Sleep or appetite problems.
  - Persistent feelings of sadness, anxiety or emptiness.
  - Constant fatigue or loss of motivation.

3. Support measures
  - **Well-being programmes**: Facilities can set up programmes to support employee wellbeing, such as stress management workshops or group therapy sessions.

- **Relaxation areas**: Areas dedicated to relaxation or meditation can help staff to unwind during their breaks.
- **Supervision and mentoring**: Allowing staff to discuss their experiences and feelings with a supervisor or mentor can be beneficial.

4. Training and awareness-raising
- Provide regular training on recognising the signs of mental distress.
- Raising staff awareness of the importance of looking after their own mental health and that of their colleagues.

5. Create a culture of support
- Fostering an environment where professionals feel safe to discuss their concerns or feelings openly.
- Encourage staff to seek help when they feel they need it, without fear of stigmatisation.

6. Resources available
- In-house mental health services.
- Telephone helplines or employee assistance programmes.
- Support groups or therapy workshops.

The mental well-being of healthcare professionals is a crucial issue, not only for their own health but also for the quality of the care they provide. Medical establishments need to recognise and actively address this issue, putting in place appropriate support measures and creating an environment where mental wellbeing is valued.

# Building a balance work-life

Work-life balance is a major issue for many healthcare professionals. The demanding nature of the medical sector, combined with the responsibility of caring for patients, can quickly swallow up personal life. Yet this balance is essential for general well-being, job satisfaction and quality of care. Here are some strategies for building and maintaining that balance.

1. Recognising the importance of balance
   - **Health and well-being**: Prolonged imbalance can lead to stress, fatigue and mental health problems.
   - **Professional efficiency**: Rest and disconnection are essential for recharging batteries and ensuring optimum performance at work.

2. Set clear limits
   - **Working hours**: As far as possible, try to keep to fixed hours. If you have to work overtime, make sure it is the exception rather than the rule.
   - **Communication**: Establish clear rules for professional communication outside working hours.

3. Time management and planning
   - **Priorities**: Define what is essential in your work and in your personal life and focus on these.
   - **Planning**: Use planning tools, such as diaries or applications, to manage your time effectively.

4. Delegating and asking for help
   - **At work**: If certain tasks can be entrusted to others, don't hesitate to delegate.
   - **At home**: Share domestic responsibilities with family members or consider outsourcing certain tasks, such as cleaning.

5. Taking time for yourself
- **Activities**: Find activities that relax you and help you decompress.
- **Holidays**: Make sure you take regular time off to rest and recharge your batteries.

6. Regular re-evaluation
- **Evaluation**: Take time every few months to reflect on your work-life balance and adjust accordingly.
- **Feedback**: Talk to your friends and colleagues to get feedback on your balance and any areas for improvement.

7. Adopt a flexible mentality
- **Adaptability**: Circumstances change, and you may need to adjust your balance to suit new situations.
- **Letting go**: Accept that everything can't always be perfect and learn to let go of the less essential elements.

Striking a work-life balance in the medical field requires ongoing effort and regular introspection. Each professional needs to find their own balance, based on their needs and priorities. By investing time and energy in this balance, healthcare professionals can not only improve their own well-being, but also the quality of the care they provide.

# Chapter 9:
# INTERACTION WITH
# VARIOUS PATIENT POPULATIONS

## Working with children in radiology

### • Distraction and calming techniques

In the medical setting, and more specifically in medical imaging, patients may experience anxiety, pain or discomfort. Distraction and calming techniques are valuable tools for reducing these unpleasant sensations and improving the patient experience. They are particularly useful during long or potentially uncomfortable examinations.

1. Why use distraction techniques and of appeasement?

- **Reducing anxiety**: Medical procedures can be stressful. Distraction helps to take the patient's attention away from their anxiety.
- **Reducing the perception of pain**: Distraction can reduce the perception of pain by occupying the mind elsewhere.
- **Facilitating cooperation**: A patient who is relaxed and distracted is often more cooperative, making the examination run more smoothly.

2. Distraction techniques

- Visual:
    - Use of relaxing videos or images.
    - Observation of moving or luminous objects.

- Hearing:
    - Listen to soothing music or natural sounds (such as the sound of rain or waves).
    - Listening to stories.
- Tactile:
    - Use of soft or textured toys.
    - Therapeutic touch techniques.
- Mental:
    - Guided breathing techniques.
    - Meditation or visualisation.
    - Word games and riddles to keep your mind occupied.

## 3. Soothing techniques
- Physical contact:
    - A simple caress or reassuring touch can have a calming effect.
    - Gently massaging certain areas (such as the hands) can be relaxing.
- Communication:
    - Speak calmly to the patient, explaining the steps in the procedure.
    - Actively listen to patients' concerns and reassure them.
- Breathing techniques:
    - Encourage the patient to take long, deep, regular breaths.
    - Guided breathing can help calm the heart rate and reduce anxiety.
- Environment:
    - Use soft lighting.
    - Ensure a comfortable room temperature.
    - Limit loud or unexpected noise.

## 4. Staff training and awareness
It is crucial that staff are trained and made aware of how to use these techniques. Correct application can make the

difference between a traumatic patient experience and a positive one.

Distraction and calming techniques are essential tools in the medical field, helping to improve patient comfort and experience. However, they require appropriate training and implementation tailored to each individual's needs and situation.

## • **Understanding the specific needs of children**

Working with children in a medical environment, and more specifically in medical imaging, requires an in-depth understanding of their specific needs. Children are not simply "little adults". They have unique reactions, emotions and needs that may vary according to their age, development and previous experiences.

1. Recognising age and development
   - Infants:
     - Can be calm when cradled or fed.
     - They respond well to gentle touch and soothing voices.
   - Toddlers (1-3 years):
     - Opposition phase, may be reluctant to follow instructions.
     - Toys or distractions can be useful.
     - Understand the concept of "pretend play" to explain procedures.
   - Pre-school (3-6 years):
     - Begin to understand simple explanations.
     - Stories or analogies can help explain procedures.
   - Primary school (6-12 years):
     - Need to know what's going to happen and why.
     - They may ask many questions to reassure themselves.

- They often want to be involved or informed.
- Teenagers (aged 12 and over):
  - They want to be treated with respect, not like young children.
  - The importance of confidentiality and autonomy.

2. Managing fear and anxiety
- **Age-appropriate communication**: Use age-appropriate language and explanations.
- **Distractions**: Books, toys, videos or music can help to distract the child during the procedure.
- **Presence of parents**: The presence of a parent or relative can often soothe a child. However, it is essential to guide parents on how to assist and reassure their child.

3. Physical needs
- **Size and shape**: Equipment and techniques must be adapted to children's size and shape.
- **Sensitivity**: Children may be more sensitive to pain or discomfort, requiring adjustments or the use of soothing techniques.

4. Respecting children
- **Autonomy**: Even when they're young, it's essential to recognise children's need for autonomy. Ask them for their opinion whenever possible.
- **Confidentiality**: Respect the child's privacy, even in the presence of parents.

5. Preparation and follow-up
- **Prepare in advance**: Explain to the child (and parents) what is going to happen before the procedure. This can help reduce anxiety.

- **Debriefing**: After the test, take the time to talk to your child, congratulate them on their bravery and answer any questions they may have.

Understanding and responding to the specific needs of children in medical imaging is essential to ensure quality care and a positive experience for the child and their family. This requires patience, empathy and specific training for healthcare professionals.

# Working with the elderly

## • Understanding common problems such as dementia

Dementia is a growing challenge due to ageing demographics in many countries. For medical imaging assistants, it is crucial to understand dementia and have the skills to effectively manage patients with this condition. This chapter explores the nature of dementia, how it affects the patient and strategies for appropriate management in medical imaging.

1. What is dementia?
   - Definition and types:
     - Dementia is not a specific disease. It is a general term for a decline in cognitive ability severe enough to interfere with daily life.
     - Alzheimer's disease, vascular dementia, Lewy body dementia, etc.
   - Common symptoms:
     - Memory loss, communication difficulties, loss of judgement, confusion, disorientation.

2. Impact on medical imaging experience
- **Unpredictable behaviour**: A patient with dementia may react differently from one day to the next.
- **Increased sensitivity**: Noises, lights or simply a change of environment can trigger anxiety or agitation.
- **Difficulty following instructions**: Patients may not understand or may quickly forget simple instructions.

3. Management strategies
- Create a calm environment:
    - Reduce excessive stimuli such as loud noises.
    - Use soft lighting where possible.
- Clear, simple communication:
    - Speak slowly and clearly.
    - Use short sentences and simple instructions.
    - Avoid medical jargon.
- Use validation techniques:
    - Rather than constantly correcting the patient, enter their world. If a patient is looking for her deceased husband, rather than saying "he passed away," we might say, "Tell me more about your husband."
- Presence of a relative:
    - Having a family member or carer with the patient during the procedure can have a calming effect.
- Distraction techniques:
    - Soothing music, relaxing images or simply talking about something the patient likes can divert their attention from the stressful aspects of the examination.
- Flexibility:
    - Be prepared to adapt to the situation. If one method doesn't work, try another.

4. Staff training and awareness
- **Specific training**: Staff should receive training in the management of patients with dementia, including understanding the condition, effective communication and techniques for dealing with challenging behaviour.
- **Simulations**: Organise simulation sessions where staff can practise scenarios with dementia 'patients' (actors or trained staff).

Caring for patients with dementia in medical imaging is a challenge that requires patience, understanding and training. By understanding the condition and adapting the approach to care, care assistants can help make the experience as positive and stress-free as possible for the patient and their family.

## • **Assistive technology for reduced mobility**
The care of patients with reduced mobility in medical imaging is a fundamental responsibility of the nursing auxiliary. These patients require specific approaches to ensure their safety, comfort and the quality of the images obtained. This chapter deals with the essential techniques and recommendations for assisting these patients during imaging procedures.

1. Understanding reduced mobility
- Different types of limitations:
- Paralysis
- Muscle weakness
- Balance disorders
- Orthopaedic problems
- Post-operative restrictions
- Fatigue due to chronic illness

2. Initial assessment
- Patient's medical history:
- Knowing the cause of the limitation will help determine the best approach.
- Patient's level of mobility:
- Can the patient walk on their own, with assistance, or not at all?
- Does he use mobility aids such as a cane, walker or wheelchair?

3. Assistance techniques
- Transfers:
    - **Standing to standing**: Support the patient by the trunk or waist.
    - **Examination table chair**: Use of transfer boards, glides or lifting aids.
    - **Wheelchair to examination table**: Make sure the wheelchair brakes are engaged and use a transfer board if necessary.
- Positioning on the examination table:
    - Use cushions and pillows for support.
    - Make sure the patient is stable and comfortable.

4. Specialised equipment
- **Patient lifts:** Mechanical devices that can help lift and move heavy or uncooperative patients.
- **Transfer board:** A flat, solid board that helps to slide the patient from one surface to another.

5. Communication with the patient
- **Explain each step**: Tell the patient what you are going to do before you do it.
- **Listening to the patient's concerns**: It is essential to understand the patient's limitations and any pain they may be experiencing.

6. Security
- **Proper lifting techniques**: To avoid injury, it is crucial to lift using the legs, not the back.
- **Getting help**: For heavier patients or those requiring special attention, always ask for extra help.
- **Avoid slips and falls**: Make sure floors are dry, use non-slip footwear and remove potential obstacles.

Assisting patients with reduced mobility requires patience, empathy and appropriate training. The nursing auxiliary plays an essential role in ensuring that these patients receive quality care while preserving their dignity and comfort. The right techniques and equipment ensure the safety and well-being of both patient and healthcare professional.

# Patients with special needs: disabilities, anxiety disorders, etc.

In medical care, every patient is unique, and some require special attention and care because of their specific needs. Understanding and managing these needs is essential to ensure the safety, comfort and respect of all patients during imaging procedures.

1. Patients with physical disabilities
- Disability assessment:
- Type of disability (paraplegia, quadriplegia, amputation, etc.)
- Level of mobility
- Equipment needs (wheelchairs, prostheses, etc.)
- Transfer and assistance techniques:
- Adapting transfer techniques
- Use of specialised equipment
- Communication:

- Talking directly to the patient and not to the carer
- Ask the patient how they would like to be helped

## 2. Patients with sensory disabilities
- Hearing impairment:
- Use of sign language, if possible
- Provide written instructions
- Ensuring good lighting for lip-reading
- Visual impairment:
- Describing procedures and the environment
- Physically guide the patient if necessary

## 3. Anxiety and other psychological disorders
- Recognising signs of anxiety:
- Sweating, trembling, rapid breathing, etc.
- Soothing techniques:
- Deep breathing
- Soothing music or white noise
- Empathetic communication:
- Reassuring the patient
- Explain each stage

## 4. Cognitive disorders
- Dementia, Alzheimer's, etc:
- Use short, clear sentences
- Making eye contact
- Repeat instructions if necessary
- Patients with autism spectrum disorders:
- Avoid excessive sensory stimuli (bright lights, loud noises)
- Provide clear and concise instructions
- May require specific planning for the timing of examinations

## 5. Paediatric patients
- Use of distraction techniques:

- Toys, stories, videos
- Explain the procedure to their level of understanding
- Include parents or guardians in the procedure:

Caring for patients with special needs in medical imaging requires a tailored, well-informed and empathetic approach. The nursing auxiliary must be equipped with the skills and knowledge necessary to meet these needs while ensuring the safety and effectiveness of imaging procedures.

# Chapter 10:
# INCIDENT MANAGEMENT
# AND COMPLEX SITUATIONS

## Procedures
## in the event of a radiological incident

Radiological incidents, although rare, can occur in any environment where medical imaging equipment is used. It is imperative that staff, including healthcare assistants, understand and follow clear protocols in the event of an incident to minimise the risks and ensure the safety of the patient and the team.

1. Definition of a radiological incident
   - **Unexpected exposure**: Any situation where an individual is exposed to radiation without medical necessity or in excess of expected levels.
   - **Equipment failure**: A malfunction of the imaging equipment that could lead to excessive exposure.

2. Immediate action
   - **Stopping exposure**: If possible, stop the machine immediately or move the patient away from the source of radiation.
   - **Ensure patient safety**: Check the patient's condition and administer first aid if necessary.
   - **Isolate the area**: If the equipment is the source of the problem, isolate the area to avoid any further exposure.

3. Notification
   - **Inform the hierarchy**: Immediately inform the radiologist in charge and the department manager.

- **Report to the radiation protection team**: they will assess the level of exposure and recommend corrective measures.

4. Assessment of the incident
   - **Document the incident**: Record all relevant details of the incident, including the date, time, patient involved, equipment used and circumstances surrounding the incident.
   - **Measuring exposure**: If possible, estimate the amount of radiation to which the patient or staff has been exposed.

5. Consequence management
   - **Medical consultation**: In certain cases, the patient or exposed personnel may need a medical assessment to determine the possible consequences of exposure.
   - **Equipment repair**: If faulty equipment is the cause of the incident, ensure that it is repaired or replaced before it is used again.

6. Preventive measures
   - **Ongoing training**: Ensure that all staff are regularly trained in radiological safety protocols.
   - **Regular equipment maintenance**: To prevent failures, make sure that equipment is regularly maintained and inspected.

7. Communication
   - **Inform the patient**: Explain the incident to the patient in a transparent way, its potential consequences and the steps to be taken.
   - **Internal communication**: Inform all departmental staff of the incident, the causes identified and the measures taken to avoid a recurrence.

Appropriate management of radiological incidents is crucial to ensuring the safety of patients and medical imaging staff. Proper training, clear protocols and open communication are essential to minimise risks and effectively manage any incidents that do occur.

# Managing reactions contrast agents

Contrast agents are often used in medical imaging to improve the visualisation of internal body structures. Although they are generally well tolerated, some patients may experience adverse reactions. It is therefore essential that care assistants and all medical staff are trained to recognise and manage these reactions.

1. Introduction to contrast agents
   - **Definition and types**: Iodine for computed tomography (CT), gadolinium for magnetic resonance imaging (MRI), etc.
   - **Route of administration**: Oral, intravenous, etc.

2. Common reactions to contrast agents
   - Mild reactions:
   - Feeling hot or cold
   - Metallic taste in the mouth
   - Mild nausea
   - Moderate reactions :
   - Hives or rash
   - Itching
   - Hot flushes
   - Serious reactions :
   - Breathing difficulties
   - Angioedema (swelling of the face or throat)
   - Hypotension
   - Anaphylactic shock

3. Procedures in the event of a reaction
- Mild reactions:
- Reassure the patient.
- Keep an eye on it until symptoms resolve.
- Moderate reactions :
- Stop administration of the contrast agent immediately.
- Administer an antihistamine if necessary.
- Monitor the patient closely.
- Serious reactions :
- Stop administration of the contrast agent.
- Call for emergency medical assistance.
- Administer adrenaline in the event of anaphylactic shock, in accordance with established protocols.
- Ensure a clear airway and, if necessary, start cardiopulmonary resuscitation.

4. Preventing reactions
- **Patient history**: Always ask the patient if they have ever had a reaction to a contrast agent or if they have any known allergies.
- **Premedication**: In certain cases, anti-allergic premedication may be administered to reduce the risk of a reaction.
- **Continuous monitoring**: Monitor the patient during and after administration of the contrast agent to detect any signs of reaction quickly.

5. Communication with the patient
- **Inform the patient**: Before administration, explain to the patient any common sensations they may experience.
- **Reassure the patient**: If a reaction occurs, keep the patient informed of what you are doing to manage the situation.

Rapid recognition and appropriate management of reactions to contrast agents are essential to ensure patient safety. Caregivers, although not substitutes for healthcare professionals in the administration of drugs or the management of serious emergencies, play a key role in monitoring and supporting patients during these procedures. Proper training and clear communication are the keys to successful care.

# Working with the team
# in the event of a medical emergency

Medical emergencies can occur at any time in radiology. Whether it's an allergic reaction to a contrast agent, respiratory distress or another unexpected event, rapid, coordinated and effective intervention by the whole team is crucial. Nursing assistants, in collaboration with radiology technicians, radiologists and nurses, play an essential role in ensuring patient safety.

1. Recognising emergency signs
   - **Continuous monitoring**: healthcare assistants must be trained to recognise abnormal vital signs, respiratory distress, pain or discomfort in the patient.
   - **Communication with the patient**: Ask the patient about his or her condition, check regularly on the patient's well-being during the examination.

2. First answer
   - **Alert**: If a medical emergency is suspected, other team members must be alerted immediately.
   - **First aid**: Pending specialist care, provide basic first aid, such as CPR (cardiopulmonary resuscitation) if necessary.

3. Working with the team
- **Role of the radiology technician**: Interrupt the examination, assist with emergency procedures, be in charge of emergency equipment.
- **Role of the radiologist**: Assessing the patient, making clinical decisions, prescribing medication or additional procedures.
- **Nurses' role**: administering medication, monitoring vital signs, supporting the medical team.

4. Emergency protocols
- **Know the protocols**: Every radiology department must have clearly established emergency protocols that every member of the team, including nursing assistants, must be familiar with.
- **Regular training**: Emergency training and simulations can help the team to be prepared and coordinated in the event of a real event.

5. After the emergency
- **Debriefing**: Once the situation has stabilised, it is essential to discuss the event with the whole team to assess what went well and identify areas for improvement.
- **Emotional support**: Medical emergencies can be stressful for staff. Offering support, such as group discussions or psychological assistance, can be beneficial.

Healthcare assistants are an integral part of the radiology team, and their role in a medical emergency is vital. Although they are not responsible for clinical decisions, their vigilance, speed of response and ability to work as part of a team are essential to ensure patient safety. Ongoing training, good communication and an understanding of emergency protocols are key to managing these situations effectively.

# Chapter 11:
# BREAST INTEGRATION
# THE MEDICAL TEAM

## Understanding the role
## of each team member

Radiology is a medical field that requires close collaboration between various professionals. Each member of the team has a specific role to play in ensuring that examinations run smoothly and patients receive optimum care. Understanding each person's role allows for better coordination and quality care.

1. The radiologist
  - **Diagnosis and interpretation**: The radiologist is a medical specialist who interprets X-ray images to make a diagnosis.
  - **Therapeutic decisions**: On the basis of the images, the radiologist may recommend surgery, treatment or further tests.
  - **Interventional procedures**: Some radiologists are also trained to carry out image-guided procedures such as biopsies.

2. The radiology technician
  - **Equipment operation**: They ensure that the machines are working properly and handle the equipment to obtain the best possible images.
  - **Patient positioning** : Positions the patient appropriately for the examination.
  - **Radiation protection**: Ensures that safety protocols are followed to minimise exposure to radiation.

3. The orderly
- **Preparing the patient**: Prepares the patient for the examination, ensures their comfortability and meets their needs during the examination.
- **Assistance during the examination**: Helps position the patient, gives instructions and monitors the patient's condition.
- **Post-examination support**: Monitor the patient after the examination, especially if contrast agents have been used.

4. The radiology nurse
- **Administration of drugs and contrast products**: Prepares and administers contrast agents or other necessary drugs.
- **Clinical monitoring**: Monitors the patient's vital signs and intervenes in the event of a reaction or emergency.
- **Patient education**: Informs the patient about the procedure, possible risks and post-examination care.

5. Other specialists
- **Surgeons, oncologists, etc.** Work closely with the radiologist to discuss the results of the images and define the best way to manage the patient.

The effectiveness of radiology care depends on the synergy between all the members of the team. Complementary skills ensure that the patient receives the best possible care, from preparation to interpretation of results and therapeutic recommendations. For nursing assistants, understanding the role of each member is essential if they are to integrate harmoniously into the team and contribute to the overall mission of the radiology department.

# Cultivating good inter-professional relations

Medical imaging is a field that relies on collaboration and communication between various professionals. Cultivating good inter-professional relationships is essential to ensuring optimal patient care and smooth running of services. Here are some strategies and considerations for achieving this:

1. Recognise the value of each team member
   - **Mutual respect**: Every role, whether radiologist, radiology technician, nursing auxiliary or nurse, is crucial to the smooth running of procedures. Respecting each other's skills and contributions strengthens team cohesion.

2. Open and honest communication
   - **Regular exchanges**: Organise team meetings to discuss cases, share feedback and address challenges.
   - **Constructive feedback**: When there are problems or misunderstandings, deal with them constructively, avoiding blame.

3. Interprofessional training
   - **Learning together**: Organising training sessions where different professionals can learn from each other.
   - **Simulations of real-life situations**: Practical exercises in which several professionals work together on simulated cases can reinforce mutual understanding.

4. Understanding other people's issues and constraints
- **Observation days**: Spend a day with another professional to better understand their role and daily challenges.
- **Open discussion**: Encouraging the sharing of experiences and concerns in a spirit of collaboration.

5. Promoting collaboration in patient care
- **Joint planning**: Discussing complex cases as a team to develop collaborative care plans.
- **Post-procedure reflections**: After an examination or procedure, take time to discuss what went well and areas for improvement.

6. Encouraging a culture of respect and support
- **Celebrate success**: Recognising and celebrating the team's achievements boosts morale and cohesion.
- **Support in difficult situations**: In an emergency or stressful situation, offering emotional support to colleagues is crucial.

7. Developing conflict resolution skills
- **Proactive management**: Tackling tensions or disagreements before they escalate.
- **Mediation**: If necessary, use a mediator to facilitate communication and problem-solving.

Cultivating good inter-professional relationships is essential to the delivery of quality radiology care. By fostering a culture of respect, communication and collaboration, not only do patients benefit from optimal care, but the working environment also becomes more pleasant and productive for everyone.

# Effective communication
# for a better patient flow

Patient flow" refers to the smooth, coordinated flow of a patient through the various stages of a service or procedure. In radiology, efficient patient flow is crucial to guaranteeing quality of care, reducing waiting times and optimising the use of resources. Communication plays a key role in achieving this. Here's how effective communication can improve patient flow in radiology.

1. Making an appointment and preparing the patient
   - **Coordination with referring doctors**: Clear communication with referring doctors helps us to understand the specific needs of each case.
   - **Patient information**: Give the patient clear instructions on the preparation required, any contraindications, how the examination is to be carried out, etc.

2. Welcoming the patient to the ward
   - **Internal communication**: Ensuring a smooth link between reception, technicians and radiologists to notify the arrival of a patient.
   - **Patient orientation**: Informing patients about the progress of their visit, the next steps and any waiting times.

3. During the examination
   - **Clear instructions**: The technician must clearly communicate to the patient what is expected of him/her during the examination (e.g. hold his/her breath).
   - **Real-time updates**: Inform the radiologist of any changes or concerns during the examination.

4. Post-review communication
- **Patient feedback**: Although the radiologist is generally in charge of the interpretation, the technician can reassure the patient about what will happen next and tell them when and how they will receive their results.
- **Transmission of images and reports**: Ensuring rapid and secure transmission of results to referring doctors for immediate treatment.

5. Managing emergency or unforeseen situations
- **Alert communication**: In the event of an anomaly or situation requiring rapid intervention, have clear protocols for alerting the right people.
- **Coordination with other departments**: For example, if a pathology is discovered that requires urgent surgery, effective communication with the department concerned is crucial.

6. Feedback and continuous improvement
- **Team meetings**: Organise regular meetings to discuss patient flow, identify bottlenecks and seek solutions.
- **Patient feedback**: Encourage feedback from patients to understand their experience and identify areas for improvement.

Effective communication is one of the pillars of optimised patient flow in radiology. Not only does it improve patient care, it also reduces stress for professionals, optimises resources and, ultimately, increases overall satisfaction. In an environment as dynamic and technological as radiology, investing in communication tools and training is essential.

# Chapter 12:
# LEGAL ASPECTS
# AND RESPONSIBILITIES

## Understanding the laws
## and regulations in radiology

As a branch of medicine, radiology is closely regulated by laws and regulations to guarantee the safety of patients and professionals, and to ensure optimum quality of care. These laws and regulations may vary from country to country and region to region, but they are generally based on common principles.

1. Introduction to regulatory issues
   - **Background**: Evolution of regulations in the face of technological advances and ethical challenges.
   - **The main players**: National and international organisations that define and supervise standards.

2. Radiation protection
   - **Protection standards**: Radiation exposure limits, inspection intervals, compulsory protective devices, etc.
   - **Personnel protection**: Dosimetry, personal protective equipment and other measures.
   - **Patient protection**: Justification of examinations, dose optimisation, compliance with protocols.

3. Equipment quality and safety
   - **Approval of machines**: Procedure for the marketing and inspection of X-ray equipment.
   - **Maintenance and periodic checks**: maintenance protocols, traceability and archiving obligations.

4. Staff training and accreditation
- **Skill levels**: Requirements for practising radiology, depending on the role (radiologist, technician, nursing assistant, etc.).
- **Continuing training**: Obligation to update knowledge, validation of skills, refresher courses.

5. Ethics and informed consent
- **Patients' rights**: Information, consent, refusal of examination, access to images and reports.
- **Confidentiality rules**: management and sharing of medical data, rights and obligations of professionals.

6. Radiology research
- **Clinical trials and studies**: Legal framework for conducting clinical trials involving radiation.
- **Innovations** : Assessment and approval process for new technologies.

7. Management of radiological incidents and accidents
- **Reporting incidents** : When and how to report an incident? To whom should it be reported?
- **Accident management**: Intervention protocols, medical care, responsibilities.

8. Interaction with other regulations
- **Teleradiology**: Specific rules relating to the practice of remote radiology.
- **Waste management**: Safe disposal of radiological waste.

Understanding the laws and regulations governing radiology is essential for any professional working in this field. Not only do they guarantee the safety of patients and professionals, they also ensure public confidence in this branch of medicine. A good knowledge of the rules and regular updating are therefore crucial if you are to practise ethically and professionally.

# Documentation and keeping medical records

Medical documentation is a fundamental element in ensuring continuity of care, facilitating communication between healthcare professionals and guaranteeing patient safety. Rigorous maintenance of medical records is not only a legal requirement, it is also essential for the diagnosis, treatment and follow-up of patients.

1. Introduction to the importance of medical records
   - **History**: From handwriting to digitisation.
   - **Medical and legal issues**: why accurate documentation is essential.

2. Composition of a radiology medical file
   - **Administrative data**: patient identity, contact details, insurance, etc.
   - **Medical history**: medical conditions, current treatments, allergies, etc.
   - **Reasons for consultation**: Reasons, symptoms, specific requests.
   - **Examinations carried out**: Type, date, observations, images.
   - **Radiological report**: interpretation of images, diagnosis, recommendations.

3. Principle of traceability
   - **Annotation of procedures**: Who carried out the examination, when, with what equipment.

- **Continuous updating**: monitoring developments, adding new exams and making any necessary changes.

4. Digitising files: benefits and challenges
   - **Radiology Information Systems (RIS)**: How they work, why they are useful.
   - **Archiving and accessibility**: data preservation, rapid search, interoperability.
   - **Security and confidentiality**: Data protection, regulations, security measures.

5. Legality and ethics of documentation
   - **Patients' rights**: access to their file, rectification, deletion.
   - **Retention**: Legal retention period for files, secure destruction.
   - **Information sharing**: With whom, when and how information can be shared.

6. Staff training and awareness
   - **Roles and responsibilities**: Who can access files, who can modify them.
   - **Ongoing training**: Regular updates on systems in place, new regulations, etc.
   -

7. Error and incident management
   - **Identifying errors**: Recognising and reporting them.
   - **Correction and follow-up**: Corrective measures, prevention of repeat offences.

8. The future challenges of radiology documentation
   - **Artificial intelligence and big data**: potential impact on record-keeping.
   - **Systems interconnection**: Facilitating the exchange of information between establishments, regions or countries.

Meticulous medical record keeping is at the heart of modern medical practice. It not only ensures the quality of care, but also protects patients and healthcare professionals. In the field of radiology, where precision is crucial, rigorous documentation is absolutely essential.

# Patients' rights
# and duties of professionals

The healthcare system, in its quest for excellence and ethics, relies heavily on the relationship between patients and healthcare professionals. This relationship is governed by a set of rights and duties designed to protect the patient while enabling professionals to provide the best possible care. Here is a detailed exploration of these rights and duties.

1. Patients' fundamental rights
   - Right to information:
     - Understand the nature and purpose of any examination or treatment.
     - Be informed of the potential risks and benefits.
   - Right to informed consent:
     - Do not undergo any examination or treatment unless you have given your consent after being duly informed.
   - Right to confidentiality:
     - Guarantee that personal and medical information remains private.
   - Right of access to medical records:
     - See, obtain a copy of or correct your own medical records.
   - The right to dignity and respect:
     - To be treated with respect and dignity, regardless of age, gender, race, religion or other discriminatory factors.

- Right to refuse treatment:
    - The right to refuse treatment or an examination without suffering reprisals.
- Right to lodge a complaint:
    - The opportunity to report dissatisfaction or damage and obtain redress.

2. The duties of healthcare professionals
    - Duty to inform:
    - Providing clear, accurate and understandable information to patients.
    - Duty of competence:
    - Provide ongoing training to ensure that skills and knowledge are kept up to date.
    - Duty of confidentiality:
    - Protecting patients' personal and medical information.
    - Duty of care:
    - Providing quality care, based on patient needs and best available practice.
    - Duty of humanity:
    - Treat every patient with respect, dignity and compassion.
    - Duty to cooperate:
    - Working with other professionals to ensure multidisciplinary care.
    - Duty of care:
    - Report any incidents or adverse events related to care.
    - Ethical duty:
    - Adhere to a code of ethics and act in the best interests of the patient.

3. The interaction between patients' rights and professionals' duties
    - Navigating complex situations:
    - Cases where patients' rights conflict with professional duties.

- Training and awareness-raising:
- The importance of continuing education on medical ethics, patients' rights and professional responsibilities.

4. Consequences of non-compliance with rights and duties
- Legal implications:
  - Possible sanctions in the event of negligence, professional misconduct or breach of confidentiality.
- Professional repercussions:
  - Impact on reputation, professional licence or career.
- Consequences for the patient:
  - Physical, emotional or psychological harm.

Mutual respect for the rights of patients and the duties of professionals is essential for creating a relationship of trust and guaranteeing high-quality care. This dynamic is at the heart of medical practice, and every professional must strive to maintain and strengthen it.

# CONCLUSION

## The growing importance radiology in medical care

Radiology is the medical speciality that uses X-rays and other forms of radiant energy to diagnose and treat disease. It has become an essential component of modern medicine, playing a crucial role in almost every aspect of medical care. Here's a look at the growing importance of radiology and how it has transformed the healthcare landscape.

1. Faster, more accurate diagnosis
   - **Real-time imaging**: Radiology allows doctors to see inside the human body in real time, offering a unique perspective that was not possible before.
   - **Early detection**: Diseases such as cancer can be detected at early stages, increasing the chances of cure and survival.

2. Reducing invasive surgery
   - **Non-invasive procedures**: Thanks to interventional radiology, many procedures that previously required surgery can now be carried out less invasively.
   - **Faster recovery**: Patients generally recover more quickly from radiological procedures than from traditional surgery.

3. Better management of chronic diseases
   - **Monitoring**: Radiology allows regular monitoring of chronic diseases, providing information on disease progression and the effectiveness of treatments.

4. Evolution with technological advances
- **Innovations**: As technology has evolved, so has radiology, with techniques such as MRI, PET scans and 3D ultrasound.
- **Augmented and virtual reality**: These technologies offer radiologists new ways of viewing and interpreting medical images.

5. Interdisciplinary
- **Collaboration with other specialities**: Radiology works closely with other medical specialities, reinforcing the importance of inter-professional communication.
- **The nerve centre of medical decisions**: In many cases, radiology provides the essential information that guides the treatment plan.

6. Training and specialisation
- **The importance of continuing education**: As radiology evolves, continuing education becomes essential to guarantee the quality of care.
- **Sub-specialties**: such as interventional cardiology and neuroradiology, offering more specialised care.

7. Raising awareness among the public and the medical profession
- **Information and education**: With the increasing use of radiology, it is essential to inform the public and healthcare professionals of the benefits and risks.

Radiology has established itself as a cornerstone of modern medical care, influencing the way diseases are diagnosed, treated and managed. Its growth and importance reflect the constant evolution of medicine and the need to provide the highest quality of care.

# Enhancing the role of the care assistant: an essential link

In the complex arena of healthcare, each role plays a vital part in ensuring the patient's well-being. Among them, the medical imaging orderly is often unknown to the general public, but his or her role is vital. This chapter aims to explore and highlight this essential role.

1. Beyond the cliché: more than just 'assistants
   - **Versatility**: The nursing auxiliary is trained to intervene in many aspects of patient care, from reception to post-examination follow-up.
   - **Practical expertise**: Although they do not directly carry out the imaging tests, their practical knowledge of the procedures is essential to ensure that they run smoothly.

2. First line of communication with the patient
   - **Reassurance and information**: The healthcare assistant is often the first person the patient meets. Their ability to inform, reassure and establish a connection is fundamental to the patient's comfort.
   - **Identifying specific needs**: Care assistants are trained to identify patients' particular needs and adapt care accordingly.

3. Working with the medical team
   - **Essential link**: They act as a bridge between patients and the rest of the medical team, passing on crucial information that can influence diagnosis and treatment.
   - **Teamwork**: Their collaboration with radiologists, technicians and other professionals ensures a smooth, efficient workflow.

4. Ensure the patient's physical and emotional well-being
  - **Preparing for the examinations**: Ensuring that the patient is correctly positioned and comfortable is essential for obtaining clear images.
  - **After the examination**: Care assistants make sure that patients feel well after the procedure, especially if a contrast agent has been used or if the patient was anxious.

5. Ongoing training for quality care
  - **Keeping up to date**: Medical technology is evolving rapidly. Care assistants must regularly update their skills to provide the best possible care.
  - **In-depth understanding**: Their training enables them to understand the complexity of equipment, procedures and patient needs.

6. Promoting the profession
  - **Institutional recognition**: Hospitals and clinics must recognise and value the crucial role of nursing assistants by offering them continuing training opportunities and career prospects.
  - **Support and respect**: In a medical environment, every role is essential. Cultivating an environment of mutual respect benefits everyone, especially patients.

Medical imaging assistants are undeniably an essential link in the healthcare chain. Valuing their role and recognising their contribution is not only necessary for the well-being of the patient, but also for the positive development of the medical sector as a whole.

# Glossary of medical terms and technical

This glossary provides a list of terms commonly used in the field of medical imaging and their respective definitions. It is intended to help nursing assistants, students and all readers to understand and familiarise themselves with professional jargon.

- **Contrast agent**: Substance injected or ingested by the patient to improve the visibility of certain structures or fluids in the body during imaging.
- **History**: Collection and analysis of a patient's medical history.
- **Angiography**: Medical imaging technique used to visualise blood vessels.
- **Anteriority:** Refers to the front of the body.
- **AP (Anteroposterior)**: An examination direction where the X-ray passes first through the anterior and then the posterior part of the body.
- **CT (computed tomography)**: A medical imaging technique that uses X-rays to obtain cross-sectional images of the body.
- **Bone densitometry**: Measures bone mineral density to assess bone strength.
- **Ultrasound:** An imaging technique that uses sound waves to produce images of internal organs.
- **Fluoroscopy**: Imaging technique that allows the movement of a contrast agent through the body to be visualised in real time.
- **MRI (Magnetic Resonance Imaging)**: An imaging technique that uses magnets and radio waves to produce detailed images of organs and tissues.
- **Laterality:** Refers to the left or right side of the body.
- **Mammography:** Medical imaging technique specifically designed to visualise breast tissue.

- **Occlusion**: Blockage or closure of a blood vessel or duct.
- **Posteriority:** Refers to the back of the body.
- **Interventional radiology**: uses imaging techniques to guide minimally invasive medical procedures.
- **Radiation protection**: Measures and procedures designed to protect individuals from radiation.
- **Scintigraphy**: Medical imaging technique that uses radiotracers to visualise specific organ functions.
- **Sonogram**: Image obtained by ultrasound.
- **Teleradiology: the** practice of remote interpretation of medical images.
- **Ventral:** Refers to the front part of the body.

This glossary is an introduction to the medical and technical terms commonly used in medical imaging. A thorough understanding of these terms will facilitate communication between healthcare professionals and improve patient care.

# Resources for continuing education

Ongoing training is essential for nursing assistants working in medical imaging. It enables them to keep abreast of the latest technological advances, best clinical practice and new regulations. Below is a list of resources for continuing education:

- Academic institutions and vocational schools :
  - Advanced courses in medical imaging.
  - Practical workshops.
  - Specialist conferences.
- Professional associations :
  - Annual conferences.
  - Seminars and workshops.
  - Publications and newsletters.
  - Online courses and webinars.
- Specialist newspapers and magazines:
  - Journal of Radiology.
  - Radiology Today.
  - Clinical Radiology.
- E-learning platforms :
  - MOOCs specific to medical imaging.
  - Sites such as Coursera, Udemy and Khan Academy offer courses in medical imaging.
  - Live and on-demand webinars.
- Simulation centres :
  - Practical training on radiology equipment.
  - Clinical case scenarios to improve patient care skills.
- Regulatory and certification bodies :
  - Mandatory training to maintain certification.
  - Regular updates on standards and directives.
- Equipment suppliers :
  - Training in the use and maintenance of new equipment.
  - Software and technology updates.

- Professional social networks :
  - Specialist groups on platforms such as LinkedIn.
  - Exchange and discuss the latest trends and research.
- Books and publications :
  - Reference books on medical imaging.
  - Practical guides and manuals.
- Mentoring :
  - Learning from experienced professionals.
  - Advice, guidance and feedback.

By investing time and resources in continuing education, medical imaging orderlies can ensure optimum patient care, while enhancing their skills and expertise. It is advisable to draw up an annual continuing education plan, and to keep abreast of opportunities available both locally and remotely.

# References and recommended reading

Medical imaging is a vast and constantly evolving field. For those who wish to deepen their knowledge, here is a list of references and recommended reading:

- Basic books :
    - Introduction to Medical Imaging: Fundamentals by Webb, Sprawls.
    - Handbook of radiology for technicians by Frank, Long, and Smith.
- Specialisation in medical imaging :
    - MRI for technicians by Westbrook.
    - Basic principles of Seeram CT scanning.
- Patient care in medical imaging :
    - Patient care in medical imaging by Romer and Sando.
    - Communication in medical imaging by Darnell.
- Radiation protection :
    - Radiation protection for technicians and radiologists by Statkiewicz Sherer, Visconti, and Ritenour.
- History of radiology :
    - Glasser's discovery of the X-ray.
- Readings on challenges and ethics :
    - Ethics in radiology by Cathey and Gaylord.
    - Psychological challenges in radiology by Mainiero and Sullivan.
- Specialist magazines :
    - Journal of diagnostic and interventional radiology.
    - Radiology.
    - European Journal of Radiology.
- Newspapers on radiology :
    - Radiology Today.
    - AuntMinnie.

- Guides for care assistants :
  - The medical imaging orderly: A practical guide by Jones and Kelly.
  - Positioning techniques for radiology technicians by Bontrager and Lampignano.
- Readings on the future of radiology :
  - The future of radiology by Dreyer and Hirschorn.
- Online resources :
  - Websites of professional societies such as the Société Française de Radiologie.
  - Online education portals such as Radiopaedia or Medscape for regular updates on technologies and case studies.

Professionals are advised to expand their reading regularly to ensure that they are up to date with the latest advances and best practices in radiology. This not only contributes to better patient care, but also to personal and professional enrichment.

www.ingramcontent.com/pod-product-compliance
Lightning Source LLC
Chambersburg PA
CBHW062318290526
45794CB00005B/1833